Clinical Decisions in Glaucoma

SECOND EDITION

TA CHEN CHANG, M.D.

Bascom Palmer Eye Institute
Department of Ophthalmology
University of Miami School of Medicine

PRADEEP RAMULU, M.D., M.H.S., PH.D.

Wilmer Eye Institute
Department of Ophthalmology
The Johns Hopkins University School of Medicine

ELIZABETH HODAPP, M.D.

Bascom Palmer Eye Institute
Department of Ophthalmology
University of Miami School of Medicine

Illustrated by
Aristomenis Thanos, M.D.

Books may be purchased in quantity at www.amazon.com.

Printed in the United States of America.

Bascom Palmer Eye Institute
900 NW 17th Street, 450N
Miami, FL 33136
tachenchang@hotmail.com
Version 11 July 2016

ISBN: 978-0692630846 (Ta Chen Chang)

10 9 8 7 6 5 4 3
1. Glaucoma 2.Clinical decisions
Second Edition

DEDICATION

To Francisco E. Fantes, M.D. (1954 – 2012)
A visionary, mentor, colleague, and dear friend.

CONTENTS

ACKNOWLEDGMENTS

The authors would like to thank –

Our friend Dr. V. Michael Patella, for his extraordinary and generous technical insights;

Our wonderful volunteer copy editors, Dr. Kateki Vinod, Dr. Andrew Camp, and Dr. Swarup Swaminathan, for their meticulous reviews and constructive criticisms;

Our spouses and children, for their patience and support;

Our colleagues in Baltimore and Miami, for their invaluable input and encouragement;

Our mentors and students, for inspiring this project;

Our patients, for their trust in our care.

PREFACE

The first edition of <u>Clinical Decisions in Glaucoma</u> was published twenty-three years ago. Since then, the principles of glaucoma management have remained the same, but much else has changed. In 1993, fundus cameras used film. Optical coherence tomography did not exist. Our medical treatments were miotics, beta-blockers, epinephrine compounds, and oral carbonic anhydrase inhibitors. Static threshold perimetry had moved into common use, but we lacked the testing algorithms and analytic tools of today. A second edition seems warranted to deal with the diagnostic and therapeutic choices available in 2016.

This edition keeps the structure of the first. It is a management manual, not a textbook. Our goal is to help the ophthalmologist or optometrist care for patients who have or may have glaucoma. We view common glaucoma as a chronic condition, one that is managed for many years in most patients.

We present first the general principles underlying our approach to glaucoma care and our overall glaucoma management scheme (Chapter 1). Next we detail what to do in the common clinical presentations suggestive of glaucoma. We do not present every possible situation, nor do we discuss every possible permutation of those situations we do present. Rather, we emphasize the common conditions and conditions for which there is specific treatment.

The most frequent findings that suggest that an individual may have glaucoma are elevated intraocular pressure or an abnormal optic disc. Less commonly a visual field abnormality or abnormal angle appearance alerts the clinician to the possibility of glaucoma. Most such patients lack symptoms, so we first describe the evaluation of an asymptomatic individual suspected of having glaucoma (Chapter 2). We do not go into great detail as to how to perform a physical examination, but we present our mental checklists of what to look for at various steps of the examination. Next we detail our method for determining if glaucoma is present based on the patient's initial findings (Chapter 3) and the management of manifest glaucoma (Chapters 4 and 5). We then present our approach to glaucoma suspects (Chapters 6 to 8). Next we deal with acutely symptomatic elevated pressure (Chapter 9) and with elevated pressure occurring in conjunction with uveitis (Chapter 10) and surgical and accidental trauma (Chapter 11). Finally we review particular management points for the more common secondary glaucomas and miscellaneous conditions associated with glaucoma (Chapter 12).

As in the first edition of this book, we have omitted extensive explanations and discussions of the various alternatives for treatment. We do not deal with all the possible complexities of clinical diagnosis and decision making. We have elected to describe what we currently think is best, based on our experience and on published information, and we try to be as explicit as possible. In our guidelines we use numbers and percentages and precise follow-up intervals. The numbers and intervals are arbitrary, but we consider them to be reasonable. We use the imperative voice frequently consistent with our view of this as a management manual.

1 GENERAL PRECEPTS

Intraocular pressure (IOP) relates to, but does not define, glaucoma. Many conditions labeled "glaucoma" have an IOP sufficiently elevated that it may produce ocular symptoms such as visual acuity loss or pain. Also included in the "glaucoma" category are cases with characteristic optic nerve damage without elevated IOP. We use the term "glaucoma" to describe a group of conditions characterized by chronic, progressive optic neuropathy which are associated with a typical pattern of retinal ganglion cell layer loss. Glaucoma may be recognized by visual field defects, changes in the optic nerve appearance, thinning of the retinal nerve fiber layer, or some combination of these findings.

The pathophysiology of chronic glaucomatous optic nerve damage has received much attention but mostly remains clinically tangential. In the future it may be possible to modify elements other than IOP that contribute to optic nerve damage. Currently, however, IOP reduction is the only established method of slowing or halting glaucomatous progression. The goal of long-term glaucoma management is to lower the IOP enough to prevent visual loss related to optic nerve damage.

Our management scheme for glaucoma is based on these general precepts:

1. The higher the IOP, the greater the risk of acquiring glaucomatous damage, and the greater the rate of glaucomatous progression.
2. There are factors other than IOP that contribute to optic nerve damage and determine an individual's susceptibility to harm from IOP, but there is, at the moment, no effective treatment for glaucoma other than IOP reduction.
3. In patients with glaucoma, lowering IOP decreases the rate of glaucomatous damage, but there is no way to know with certainty at what IOP level glaucomatous damage ceases or will be acceptably slow for a given person.
4. Every method of lowering the IOP causes side effects, costs money, and involves risk to the patient.
5. The goal of treatment for glaucoma is to lower IOP enough to preserve good vision for the lifetime of the patient while causing as few side effects and incurring as few costs as possible.

Few dispute the importance of decreasing the IOP in patients with glaucoma. However the relationship between the degree of IOP elevation and the rate of damage varies from person to person, and hence the benefit of lowering the IOP varies among individuals. For each patient, the benefit of lowering IOP should outweigh the risks and cost of the treatment.

Our two fundamental management requirements are derived from the general precepts and the chronic nature of glaucoma:

1. Glaucoma management involves balancing the risks and benefits of lowering the IOP in each patient individually.
2. Glaucoma management depends on the ability to recognize change in status over time.

Simply recognizing the presence of glaucomatous damage, particularly the earliest signs of damage, helps little in the chronic care of a patient. It is the *rate* of damage that is important. We recommend managing patients with findings suggestive of glaucoma by taking the following steps:

1. Address any treatable conditions, such as pupillary block or proliferative retinopathy, that contribute to elevated IOP. Also prophylactically treat conditions that are likely to cause elevated IOP, such as a narrow angle with high-risk features, to prevent a pathologic condition rather than dealing with it after it arises.
2. Establish a baseline by quantifying the structural and functional status of the optic nerve.
3. Decide if therapy is indicated now; if so, set a target pressure.
4. Treat the patient to achieve the target pressure. If this proves difficult, re-evaluate the chosen target pressure.
5. Follow the patient's course to see both if the IOP is controlled and if the rate of damage has decreased sufficiently.
6. Modify treatment and target pressure as indicated by the patient's course.

2 EVALUATING THE ASYMPTOMATIC PATIENT

A patient may be suspected of having glaucoma for many reasons, such as an elevated intraocular pressure (IOP), a suspicious appearance of the optic disc, an abnormal visual field finding, an abnormal angle appearance, or a combination of these factors. The objectives of the *initial* glaucoma evaluation of an asymptomatic patient, completed in one visit or over several closely-spaced visits, are as follows:

1. Address any treatable conditions that contribute to current IOP elevation or may cause future IOP elevation.
2. Establish a baseline by quantifying the structural and functional status of the optic nerve.
3. Determine if the patient has manifest glaucoma based on clinical examination, optic disc imaging, and visual field testing.
4. Decide if therapy is indicated, and, if so, set a target pressure.
5. Set an initial follow-up schedule.

The Patient with Elevated IOP

Elevated IOP – not visual symptoms – first identifies many patients who have glaucoma. Not everyone with high pressure has glaucoma, but the doctor should evaluate patients with high eye pressure and should follow up on their future courses, regardless of whether the evaluation reveals glaucoma. No clear boundary separates *elevated* from *normal* pressure; the higher the IOP, the greater the patient's likelihood to have or to develop glaucomatous optic nerve damage. It may not be sensible to divide eyes arbitrarily into those with "normal" or "high" pressure at a sharp cutoff point, but the terms "elevated pressure" and "ocular hypertension" are in common use and are unlikely to disappear soon. As an arbitrary point at which to become suspicious, the traditional definition of elevated pressure as a pressure of 22 mmHg or greater (two standard deviations above the mean in the European population)[1] serves as well as any other. Of course, we recommend that every complete ocular examination be performed with the possibility of glaucoma firmly in mind (always evaluate the optic nerve and anterior chamber), but we recommend an expanded evaluation, including gonioscopy and formal visual field/retinal nerve fiber layer assessment, for those patients whose pressure is 22 mmHg or greater.

Most patients who are found to have high pressure on routine examinations have one of the following conditions:

- Primary open angle IOP elevation (glaucoma or glaucoma suspect)
- Primary angle closure IOP elevation (glaucoma or glaucoma suspect)
- Pseudoexfoliation with IOP elevation (glaucoma or glaucoma suspect)
- Pigment dispersion with IOP elevation (glaucoma or glaucoma suspect)

The most important aspect of the evaluation of an asymptomatic individual who has elevated pressure is to identify any cause of pressure elevation for which something particular can or should be done. The less important aspect of this *initial* evaluation is deciding if glaucomatous damage already exists.

With a complete examination (including gonioscopy), clinicians can distinguish the various likely causes of high pressure and identify the occasional patient with an unusual cause. In the ordinary course of an evaluation, the history and refraction, as well as external, pupillary, motility, and anterior segment examinations, precede tonometry. When the pressure is elevated, it may be necessary to obtain additional history and reexamine the eye to look for subtle findings that may aid differential diagnosis. The salient points for each part of the evaluation follow.

History

There are two types of historical information to obtain: history related to diagnosis and history related to management decisions.

Diagnostic points –

Corticosteroid use. Oral or topical (for example, to the skin of the face) corticosteroids may elevate the IOP.

Injury. Trauma may cause damage to the outflow system which, years later, results in elevated pressure. If the patient had recent trauma or has had intraocular surgery, refer to Chapter 11.

Management points –

Family history. Glaucoma is often hereditary. If any of the patient's relatives has glaucoma, determine the severity of the disease. In our experience, a family history of severe glaucoma increases the suspicion that a patient may have a similarly severe course. The opposite, a family history of mild disease, is not as reliable a predictor.

Medical history. Patients who are severely allergic to sulfa drugs or who have renal disease are relatively poor candidates for topical or systemic carbonic anhydrase inhibitor use. Some cardiac and asthmatic respiratory problems may worsen during beta-blocker use. Vasospastic disease (migraine, Raynaud phenomenon) and low blood pressure may increase a patient's susceptibility to pressure-induced damage. A past hemodynamic crisis may explain optic nerve damage that is related to previous changes in perfusion of the optic nerve rather than to the present IOP.

Examination

Refraction. Always use the best refraction and an appropriate add for perimetry. Axial myopia probably makes the eye more susceptible to pressure-induced damage, and accompanying retinal degeneration may confound visual field evaluation. Highly hyperopic eyes are prone to develop primary angle closure.

Slit lamp examination. Pigment dispersion syndrome, pseudoexfoliation syndrome, asymptomatic inflammation, and remote and forgotten trauma may all have slit lamp findings. Examine the cornea for a Krukenberg spindle and check carefully for anterior segment inflammation. Look for iris transillumination defects, neovascularization (unusual in an asymptomatic patient), and the residua of trauma, such as iris sphincter rupture. Also look for corectopia, iris atrophy, or pseudonevus formation. After the pupil is dilated, examine the lens for pseudoexfoliation.

If the patient has had cataract surgery, the timing and nature of the procedure is relevant. First determine whether the surgery was uneventful or complicated. Following uneventful surgery, elevated IOP may be due to residual inflammation with an open angle (early postoperative period) or chronic angle closure due to uncontrolled, often low grade, inflammation (any time after surgery). Following complicated surgery, pseudoexfoliation should be suspected, and retained cortical material and secondary lens particle obstruction ruled out. If an anterior chamber intraocular lens (IOL) was implanted, note whether a patent iridotomy* is present. Also inspect and record the position of the IOL. A poorly positioned IOL either in the posterior chamber (haptic prolapsed into sulcus) or anterior chamber (poorly-sized and mobile) can cause both inflammation and elevated IOP. Increased IOP after surgery is discussed in Chapter 11.

Pachymetry. Measure the patient's central corneal thickness. We do not differentiate between measurements by contact echographic pachymeters and noncontact optical pachymeters. Central corneal thickness is useful in calculating the patient's risk of developing glaucoma if he or she is classified as a glaucoma suspect due to ocular hypertension after the initial evaluation.

Tonometry. Applanation tonometry is standard; record the time of measurement. The pressure in the two eyes rarely differs by more than 2 mmHg in normal eyes, but moderate asymmetry of pressure is common in primary open angle glaucoma. Widely disparate readings, especially if only one reading is above normal, suggest a unilateral process. In an asymptomatic patient with unilateral elevated IOP, pseudoexfoliation syndrome and old trauma are the most common diagnoses. We do not adjust IOP based on the patient's central corneal thickness.

---

* The term *iridotomy* is used through this book to refer to a hole in the iris. Unless *surgical* iridectomy is specified, we assume that an iridotomy (if recommended) will be performed with a laser.

Gonioscopy. First determine if the angle is open or closed. If the angle is open, then look for such findings as heavy pigmentation, angle recession, neovascularization, developmental anomalies, or blood in Schlemm's canal. These findings suggest particular diagnoses. If the angle is closed or very narrow, determine the type of angle closure or narrowing. Perform compression gonioscopy if unable to clearly determine the details of the iris insertion. The three general mechanisms of angle closure, illustrated in Figure 2-1, are pupillary block (common), anterior pulling (occasional), and posterior pushing (rare). Additional variants on pupillary block in traumatic, postoperative, aphakic, or pseudophakic patients are described in Chapter 11.

The distinction among different types of angle closure proceeds by first noting if there is either inflammation or some other obvious cause of angle closure other than pupillary block. Unless another diagnosis, such as an iridocorneal endothelial syndrome, rubeosis iridis, or uveitis with peripheral anterior synechiae (PAS) is clear, perform an iridotomy because it is otherwise difficult to rule out pupillary block. Management of narrow angles in individuals with normal IOP is discussed in Chapter 8.

After the iridotomy, reexamine the eye with the gonioprism. If pupillary block was present, the angle should be open or PAS should be visible. If pupillary block was absent, completion of the examination generally clarifies the cause. When the pupil is dilated, reexamine the angle and check the pressure to rule out plateau iris, which is discussed in Chapter 9.

The Patient with Abnormal Angle Appearance

When a patient has an abnormal angle appearance but does not have current angle closure, management depends on the pressure. If the pressure is elevated, proceed as discussed in previous sections. If the pressure is not elevated, determine whether the optic discs and visual fields are normal. If both are normal, proceed as discussed in Chapter 8. If either the disc or visual field is suspicious, proceed as discussed in Chapter 7.

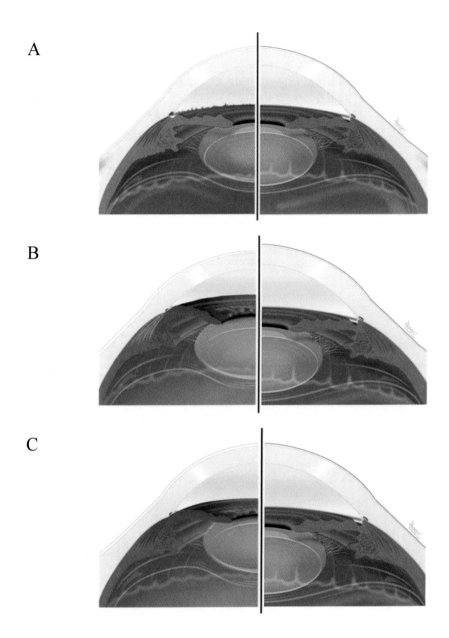

FIG 2-1. **A.** Anterior pulling angle closure, *left*; normal for comparison, *right*. Aqueous humor flows freely from the posterior to the anterior chamber. The central anterior chamber depth does not change as a result of the angle closure. **B.** Pupillary block angle closure, *left*; normal for comparison, *right*. Because of resistance to aqueous humor flow between the posterior and anterior chambers, pressure in the posterior chamber rises and aqueous humor pushes the peripheral iris forward. The anterior lens surface does not move forward, but, as shown, primary pupillary block glaucoma usually develops in smaller-than-average eyes with shallow central anterior chambers. **C.** Posterior pushing angle closure, *left*; normal for comparison, *right*. The lens moves forward and pushes the iris over the trabecular meshwork. The central anterior chamber is shallowed.

Differential Diagnostic Steps

The anterior segment examination provides the information necessary to satisfy the first two goals of the evaluation of elevated IOP, to identify specifically treatable causes of elevated pressure and to recognize if a person belongs to a particular diagnostic group (Chart 2-1).

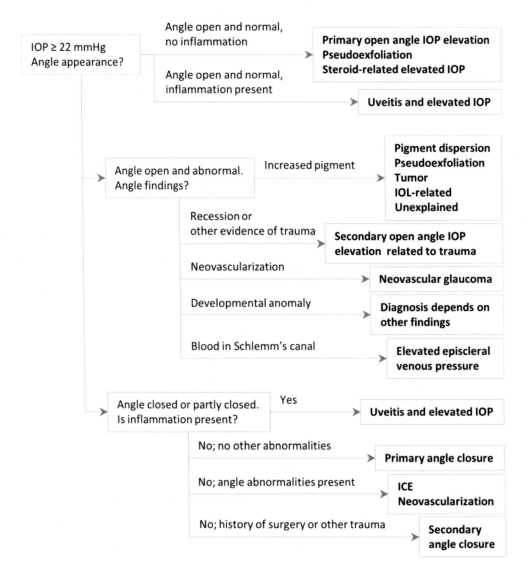

CHART 2-1. Differential diagnosis of elevated pressure in an asymptomatic eye. The majority of patients belong to one of these groups. Key – ICE (iridocorneal endothelial syndrome), IOP (intraocular pressure), IOL (intraocular lens implant).

IOP ≥ 22 mmHg, angle open and normal. In a quiet eye with normal pigment and no obvious abnormalities, the most likely diagnosis is primary open angle pressure elevation. Pseudoexfoliation with elevated pressure also generally presents in this way. It is managed the same as primary pressure elevation with a few special considerations mentioned in Chapter 12. The angle appears normal in individuals with corticosteroid-induced pressure elevation, which is also discussed in Chapter 12. If there is anterior segment inflammation, evaluate and manage the patient as described in Chapter 10.

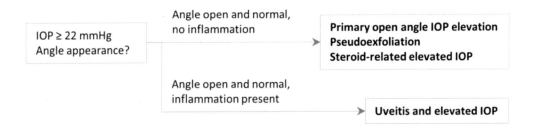

IOP ≥ 22 mmHg, angle open and abnormal –

Increased pigmentation in an open angle usually indicates either pigment dispersion syndrome or pseudoexfoliation syndrome. Pigment dispersion typically occurs in young myopic individuals, usually men, who also have Krukenberg spindles and iris transillumination defects. Pseudoexfoliation syndrome develops in older people, and the diagnosis depends on finding exfoliative material on the pupillary border and lens capsule. Both conditions are treated similarly to primary open angle pressure elevations and are discussed in Chapter 12. A secondary type of pigment dispersion occasionally develops in eyes with lens implants that chafe the posterior iris (sometimes as a part of the uveitis-glaucoma-hyphema [UGH] syndrome). Rarely, an intraocular tumor – typically a melanoma – sheds pigmented cells into the angle. If no other explanation for pigmentation is found, examine the eye carefully for tumor, especially if the pigmentation is unilateral.

Angle recession or other evidence of trauma (subluxed lens, choroidal rupture) is most often noted in patients with unilateral elevated pressure. The management of glaucoma following trauma resembles that of primary open angle glaucoma with differences discussed in Chapter 11.

Neovascularization of the anterior segment rarely causes elevated IOP without symptoms. The evaluation and management of neovascularization are discussed in Chapter 9.

Developmentally abnormal angles are occasionally noted in an asymptomatic individual with elevated pressure. Many patients' findings fall into the Axenfeld-Rieger group, but others have findings such as high iris insertions, multiple iris processes, or peculiar iris stroma that do not "fit" a specific syndrome. In the Axenfeld-Rieger group, gonioscopy may show peripheral iris atrophy, heavy uveal meshwork, and iris strands that bridge the angle and attach to or in front of Schwalbe's line, which is often thickened and anteriorly displaced. Slit lamp findings include iris atrophy and pupillary irregularity. Adult patients seen with these findings are generally treated as are those with primary open angle pressure elevation or fully developed glaucoma.

Blood in Schlemm's canal in an eye with elevated IOP may indicate elevated episcleral venous pressure. The most common causes are congenital anomalies, such as Sturge-Weber syndrome, which are associated with other visible vascular anomalies. However, in some individuals, high pressure related to acquired, asymptomatic arteriovenous shunts may develop.[2] High pressure associated with elevated episcleral venous pressure is discussed in Chapter 12.

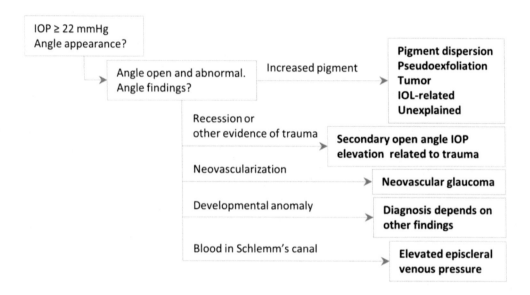

IOP ≥ 22 mmHg, angle closed or partly closed. The differential diagnosis depends on the presence or absence of anterior chamber inflammation, obvious angle abnormalities, or previous surgical or accidental trauma.

Uveitis and elevated IOP. Inflammation causes angle closure by all three of the mechanisms described in Figure 2-1. Anterior segment inflammation can result in both peripheral anterior synechiae, which pull the iris anteriorly over the trabecular meshwork, and in posterior synechiae, which seal the pupil and cause pupillary block and iris bombé. In addition, posterior segment inflammation may precipitate angle closure by rotating the ciliary body and pushing the lens forward (Figure 10-1, page 171). Evaluation and treatment are discussed in Chapter 10.

Primary angle closure. When an asymptomatic person has angle closure and elevated IOP in an unoperated eye without inflammation, the most common cause is primary chronic angle closure related to pupillary block. The first step in management is to perform an iridotomy. If the pressure falls (even if not to normal) after the iridotomy, an asymptomatic person with chronic angle closure is managed as described in Chapter 9 (page 165, Primary Acute Angle Closure – Chronic treatment). If the pressure does not decrease in an asymptomatic patient with chronic angle closure, evaluation and treatment are almost identical to that of primary open angle pressure elevation, with specific differences discussed in Chapter 12. Angle closure without other obvious abnormality that is not relieved by iridotomy is evaluated as described in Chapter 9. Angle closure in an eye that has had recent surgery or injury is discussed in Chapter 11.

Iridocorneal endothelial (ICE) syndrome. Several distinct syndromes (essential iris atrophy, Chandler syndrome, Cogan-Reese iris nevus syndrome) are associated with angle closure and may be present in an asymptomatic person with elevated pressure. They generally occur in one eye of young, usually female individuals. If typical iris findings – corectopia, iris atrophy, or pseudonevus formation – are present, the diagnosis is easy. Iridotomy does not prevent progression of the angle closure, and management resembles that of open angle IOP elevation. Particular provisos are outlined in Chapter 12.

Neovascularization is rare in this setting. It is usually associated with at least mild inflammation and is usually associated with symptoms. It is evaluated and managed as described in Chapter 9.

Secondary angle closure after surgery is discussed in Chapter 11.

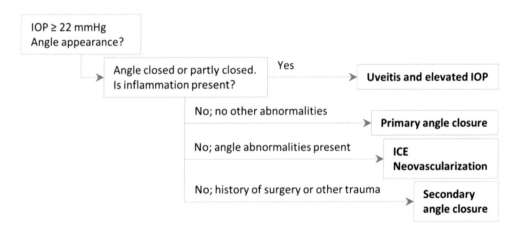

At this point in the examination, the major treatable causes of IOP elevation will have been noted. Most patients will have had no anterior segment abnormalities other than elevated pressure, and the pressure elevation is "primary" or "idiopathic." The final aspects of the initial examination, the fundus and visual field examinations, rarely contribute to the diagnosis of the type of pressure elevation, but they are the basis for establishing the stage or severity of the disease and the way in which management will proceed.

The Patient with Suspicious Optic Discs

Frequently, an asymptomatic patient with normal IOP is suspected to have glaucoma based on incidental optic disc findings. There are no pathognomonic signs for a glaucomatous disc, although certain findings, such as vertical cupping greater than 0.7 or disc margin hemorrhage, suggest acquired damage. [3, 4]

Clinical Examination

Using a slit lamp beam and a fundus lens, examine the optic disc at high magnification with the patient's pupils dilated. The slit beam defines contour better than does diffuse illumination. Indirect fundus lenses, such as the 78D or 90D lens, provide adequate anatomic details without sacrificing efficiency. However, direct lenses, such as the Hruby lens or the fundus contact lens, provide better stereopsis than do indirect lenses. Assess the color and width of the neural rim, the size and contour of the cup, and the presence or absence of notches and hemorrhages. Express to the nearest one tenth the ratio of the vertical diameter of the cup to the vertical diameter of the disc. After examining the disc, evaluate the fundus for evidence of other disease. In particular, look for old branch retinal vessel occlusions or other retinal lesions that might correspond to any field defects present.

The evaluation of suspicious optic discs is discussed in Chapter 7.

Optic Disc and Retinal Nerve Fiber Layer Imaging

The optic discs should be photographed or otherwise imaged for the sake of future comparison. The most useful photographs are stereoscopic and magnified (2x standard fundus magnification). Photographs provide a permanent color record that can be taken with the patient if he or she moves. Few clinicians can accurately capture the disc appearance on a drawing, and even the best hand drawings are less satisfactory than photographs because of the mobility of patients and the mobility and mortality of physicians. We consider photographs detailed to third order retinal vessels to be of adequate quality.

Optical coherence tomography of the circumpapillary retinal nerve fiber layer (OCT-RNFL) thickness is a useful adjunct to optic disc examination. It provides both quantitative measurements (thickness) and qualitative characterization (contour) of the RNFL, neither of which can be assessed by examination alone.

All OCT-RNFL analysis examples in this text are spectral-domain studies from the Zeiss Cirrus high definition optical coherence tomography machine (Zeiss Meditec, Inc., Dublin, California, United States of America). There are several other brands of OCT instruments available, and most operate on the same general principles and provide similar information. We consider a scan with signal strength of at least 7/10 to be adequate.

Retinal nerve fiber layer thickness (Figure 2-2). The circumpapillary RNFL thickness is analyzed as an overall average (most useful in longitudinal follow-up), in quadrants (most useful in comparison with nomograms) and in clock hours. The thickness displays are usually color-coded for patients over the age of 18 years. Values above those of 95% of the age-adjusted normal population are colored white, between the 5th and 95th percentile are colored green, between the 1st and 5th percentile are colored yellow, and below the 1st percentile are colored red. We consider a RNFL thickness analysis of adequate signal strength with any of the following features to be <u>abnormal</u>:

- Overall average below the 5th percentile (yellow or red);
- Any quadrants below the 5th percentile (yellow or red);
- Any clock hour below the 1st percentile (red).

Retinal nerve fiber layer contour (Figure 2-3). The circumpapillary RNFL contour is displayed from left to right in the order of temporal, superior, nasal, inferior and back to temporal (TSNIT graph). In patients over 18 years of age, the values are plotted against an age-adjusted nomogram with a solid line for the right eye and a dotted or broken line for the left eye. Normal TSNIT contour has tall, rounded peaks of similar heights at the inferior and superior poles and follows the overall shape of the nomogram closely. In normal fellow eyes the RNFL contours closely resemble each other. We consider a circumpapillary TSNIT RNFL contour with any of the following features to be <u>abnormal</u>:

- Any focal thinning in the superior or inferior pole, especially if the thickness is at or below the 5th percentile (yellow or red regions of nomogram);
- Any significant asymmetry between the right and left eye contour, especially if the departure is located superiorly or inferiorly.

If the contour is borderline or ambiguous, we consider the study to be abnormal.

In order of increasing likelihood of detecting glaucomatous damage, the following findings are possible:

1. Normal thickness and contour.
2. Abnormal thickness, normal contour.
3. Normal thickness, abnormal contour.
4. Abnormal thickness and contour.

Artifacts in Optical Coherence Tomography Analysis of the Circumpapillary Retinal Nerve Fiber Layer

The following scan artifacts should be ruled out by the physician when interpreting OCT-RNFL analyses (Figures 2-5 through 2-7): [5]

- Decentration
- Posterior vitreous detachment (PVD)-associated error
- Segmentation error due to misidentification of retinal landmarks
- Poor signal strength

Decentration. When the circumpapillary mire is decentered from the optic disc, the RNFL thickness in the quadrant in the direction of decentration will measure thinner, possibly with a corresponding thickening of RNFL thickness in the quadrant opposite the direction of decentration. This occurs because RNFL thickness naturally increases with proximity to the optic disc.

PVD-associated error. If the patient has a PVD and a dense Weiss ring, it can cause a small, localized signal dropout (shows up as a dark spot on the topography map), which can result in both localized thinning (usually visible in the clock hours analysis) and altered contour of the RNFL. As PVDs tend to be mobile, these defects may appear in slightly different locations on subsequent examinations.

Segmentation error due to misidentification of retinal landmarks. After the scans are acquired, the software in OCT machines identifies the inner and outer limits of the RNFL then calculates the RNFL thickness. If these limits are misidentified, such as in the presence of an epiretinal membrane or intraretinal cyst, both the RNFL thickness and contour may be misrepresented. Hence, it is important to inspect the images and the delineation marker lines to rule out segmentation error. This error can result in both artifactitious thinning and thickening of the RNFL.

Poor signal strength. This is usually related to the presence of media opacity, most commonly present on the ocular surface and/or in the lens, and less commonly in the vitreous. A decreased signal usually results in an artifactitiously thinned RNFL with preserved contour. [6, 7]

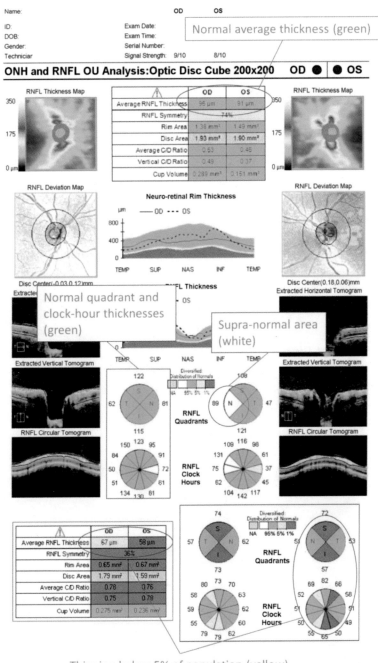

FIG 2-2. Optical coherence tomographic analysis of the circumpapillary retinal nerve fiber layer (RNFL). The RNFL analyses are presented as average, and by quadrants and clock hours. Green denotes thickness between the 5th and the 95th percentile of the normal population; yellow denote a value below the 5th percentile of the population, and red denotes thinning below the 1st percentile. Supranormal areas above the 95th percentile are colored white.

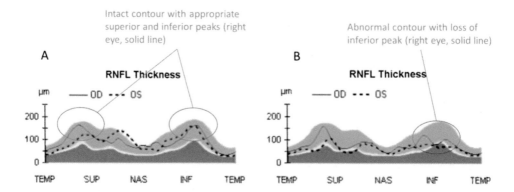

FIG 2-3. The retinal nerve fiber layer (RNFL) contour on the TSNIT graph. **A.** Normal RNFL contour has peaks at the superior and inferior poles and resembles the shape of the nomogram. **B.** Focal thinning of RNFL in the inferior pole of the right eye denoted by a dip in the thickness contour (*solid line*). The left eye has abnormal heights at both the superior and inferior poles (*dotted line*). Loss of the superior and/or inferior peak denotes abnormal contour, even if the average/quadrant thicknesses are normal.

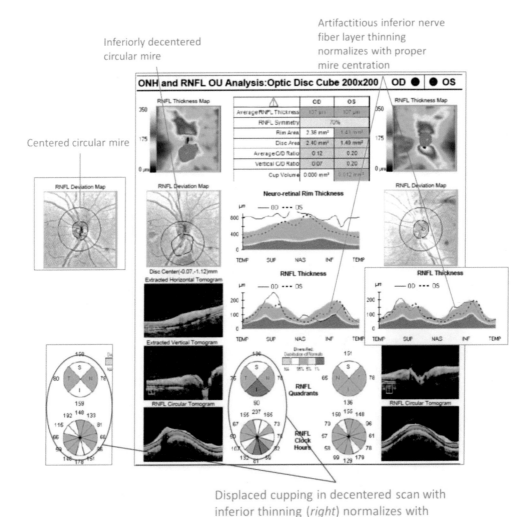

FIG 2-4. Decentration artifact. The right eye was first scanned with an inferiorly decentered circular mire and then rescanned with proper mire centration (*insets*). The decentration resulted in artifactitious inferior nerve fiber layer thinning as demonstrated on both the circular (TSNIT) thickness graph and in the quadrants and clock-hour analyses (*red ovals*). Note that nerve fiber layer thickness at the pole of the optic disc closer to the circular mire (in this example, superior) appears abnormally thick whereas the pole farther from the mire (inferior) appears abnormally thin as the retinal nerve fiber layer thickness increases closer to the optic disc.

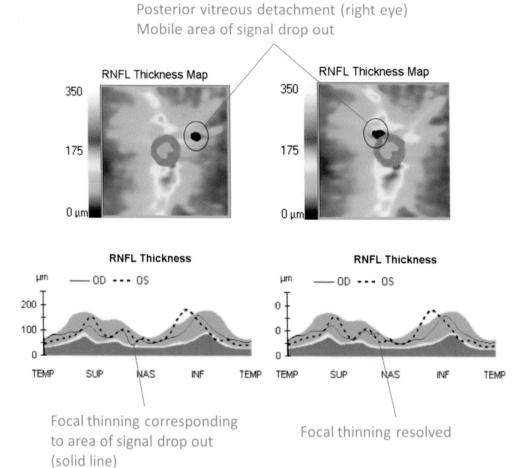

FIG 2-5. Posterior vitreous detachment-associated error. These scans are of the right eye and both were obtained during the same visit. There is a mobile area of signal drop out and corresponding focal thinning of the retinal nerve fiber layer.

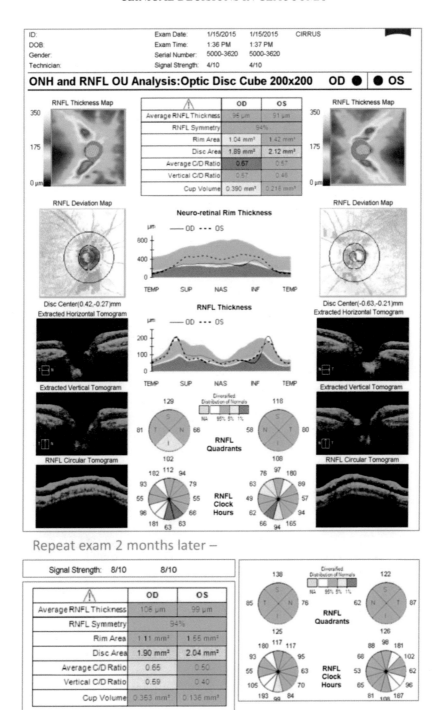

FIG 2-6. Poor signal strength resulting in artifactitious thinning of the average, quadrant and clock-hour retinal nerve fiber layer (RNFL) thickness. In the original exam dated 1/15/2015 (*top*), the signal strengths are suboptimal (4/10). On a repeat exam 2 months later (*bottom left, bottom right*), the improved signal strengths resulted in improved average, quadrant, and clock-hour RNFL thicknesses.

Normal thickness and contour. An optic disc with normal RNFL thickness and contour should have the average thickness box and all quadrants colored green or white. There should be no red clock hours. The contour should be smooth and resemble the contour of the nomogram and that of the fellow eye (Figures 2-2). These findings suggest the absence of glaucomatous optic nerve damage, [8] though sometimes glaucomatous damage may be masked due to inner and outer retina misidentification and segmentation error. [5, 9]

Abnormal thickness, normal contour (Figure 2-7). When the contour is preserved, abnormal average thickness is usually attributed to diffuse axonal loss (usually congenital) or to poor signal strength and/or scan quality due to poor media clarity. [6, 7] Highly myopic, but nonglaucomatous, eyes may show abnormal RNFL thickness with intact contour.

If the signal strength is less than 7/10, the scan should be repeated with efforts to improve scan quality. Generous ocular surface lubrication and/or pupillary dilation will often allow capture of an adequate scan. While a scan with suboptimal signal strength may not be accurate in detecting glaucomatous damage, it may still be precise enough for the longitudinal detection of change, assuming the level of media opacity remains similar.

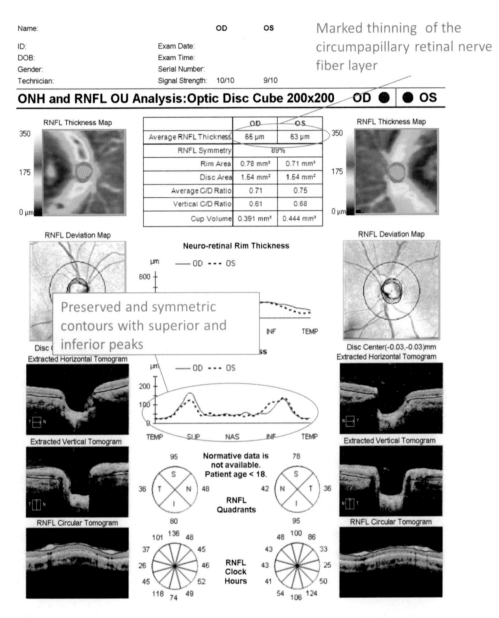

FIG 2-7. Abnormal thickness, normal contour. In this scan of a 16-year old patient, the average retinal nerve fiber layer thickness is markedly thinned (expected normal for this age range should be 100-120 microns [10]), although the contour is symmetric and intact. This patient has congenital optic nerve hypoplasia and has been followed for 2 years without progressive thinning. Note that the colored nomogram is not available in this patient who is younger than 18 years.

Normal thickness, abnormal contour (Figure 2-8). This is the least common scenario of the four presented. Occasionally, normal average, quadrant and clock hour thickness can be accompanied by a focal departure of TSNIT contour. This finding is strongly suspicious of glaucomatous damage, especially when accompanied by a corresponding visual field defect. A decentered scan or posterior vitreous detachment (PVD) can yield normal thickness but abnormal contour with focal thinning in the quadrant furthest away from center of the circular mire or in the area of the PVD, respectively (see "Artifacts in Optical Coherence Tomography Analysis of Circumpapillary Retinal Nerve Fiber Layer," page 14).

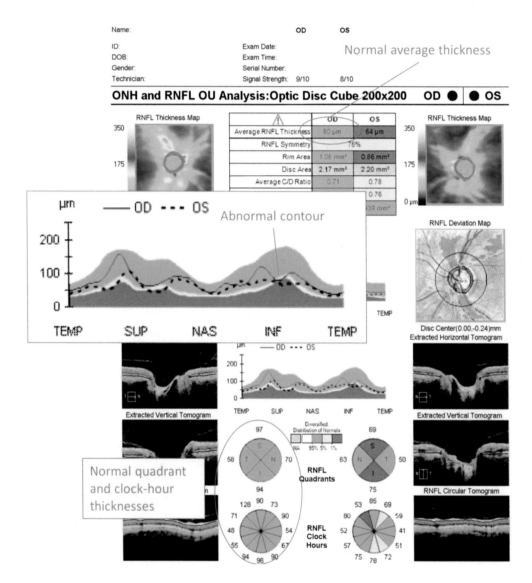

FIG 2-8. Normal thickness, abnormal contour. The average, quadrant and clock-hour thicknesses are all within normal limits. However, the contour map shows a focal dip in RNFL thickness at the inferior pole which corresponds to an early visual defect.

Abnormal thickness and contour (Figure 2-9). This is highly suspicious for glaucomatous damage. Rule out a poorly performed study with segmentation/analysis error.

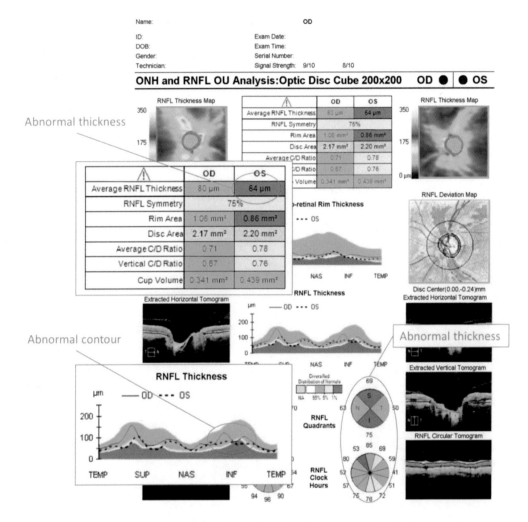

FIG 2-9. Abnormal thickness and contour. This patient's left eye demonstrates marked thinning of the average retinal nerve fiber layer as well as abnormal contour (*dotted line*).

The Patient with an Abnormal Visual Field

All complete eye examinations include some assessment of the visual field. For the many patients who are not under particular suspicion of glaucoma or other condition affecting the field, confrontation fields suffice, but patients with elevated IOP and or abnormal optic discs should have formal visual fields. It is preferable to obtain fields before ocular manipulation (tonometry, gonioscopy, or pupillary dilation). Thus, in an initial evaluation when tonometry and gonioscopy have already been completed, the fields are better tested on a separate date. If this is unrealistic, wait at least an hour to allow the corneal epithelium to recover.

We consider automated static threshold perimetry to be the standard of care in glaucoma, and we currently use a Humphrey Field Analyzer (Carl Zeiss Meditec, Inc., Dublin, California, United States of America) equipped with the STATPAC package of analyses with Guided Progression Analysis (GPA). All examples in this text are from that instrument. Extensive details about testing strategies and printout options on this and other perimeters are beyond the scope of this book but are available in standard perimetric texts. Figures 2-10 through 2-14 briefly describe the standard test program and data presentations used in this book. The three most useful analyses in glaucoma management are:

- Single Field Analysis (Figure 2-12)
- Overview (Figure 2-13)
- Guided Progression Analysis (Figure 2-14)

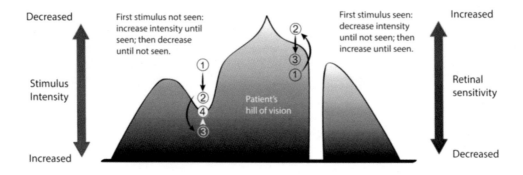

FIG 2-10. Typical strategy of threshold determination on an automated static threshold perimeter. Most perimeters increase or decrease the stimulus intensity in 4 dB steps until threshold is crossed and then move back in 2 dB steps until it is crossed again (1 dB = 0.1 log unit of attenuation of the maximum stimulus).

A

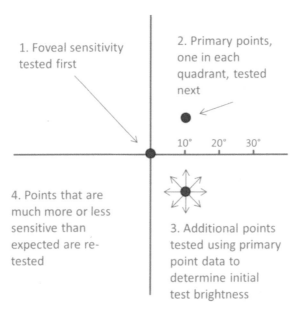

B

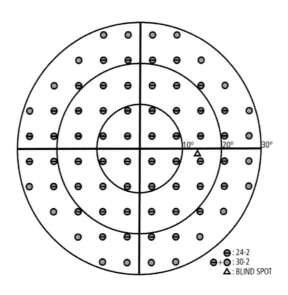

FIG 2-11. Field algorithm. **A**. General testing sequence for threshold programs on the Humphrey perimeter. **B**. Test points (right eye) on the 24-2 and 30-2 programs (reprint from *Effective Perimetry, 4th Edition*, page 29, by A. Heijl et al, 2012, Dublin, CA: Carl Zeiss Meditec, Inc. Copyright 2012 by Carl Zeiss Meditec, Inc. Reprinted with permission).

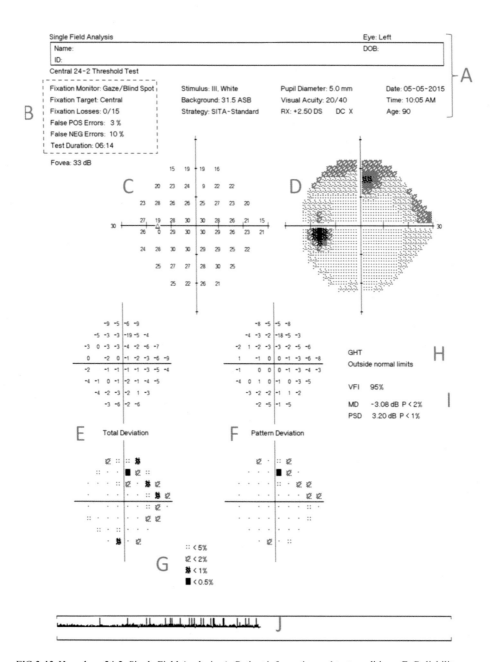

FIG 2-12. Humphrey 24-2, Single Field Analysis. **A.** Patient information and test conditions. **B.** Reliability parameters (*dash-line box*). Fixation losses, false-positive errors, and false-negative errors are discussed in the text. **C.** Test result in dB. The higher the number, the greater the visual sensitivity. **D.** Gray scale. **E.** Total deviation: the difference from normal in dB (*top*) and the likelihood that the results occurred by chance (*bottom*). **F.** Pattern deviation: the total deviation, corrected for the overall height of the hill of vision to minimize the effect of media opacity, in dB (*top*) and the likelihood that the results occurred by chance (*bottom*). **G.** Key to probability symbols. **H.** Glaucoma Hemifield Test (see page 51). **I.** Global indices. The Visual Field Index (VFI), mean deviation (MD), and Pattern Standard Deviation (PSD) are discussed in the text. **J.** Gaze tracker. A gaze deviation is recorded as a line extending upward, while inability to track gaze (e.g. a blink) is recorded as a line extending downward.

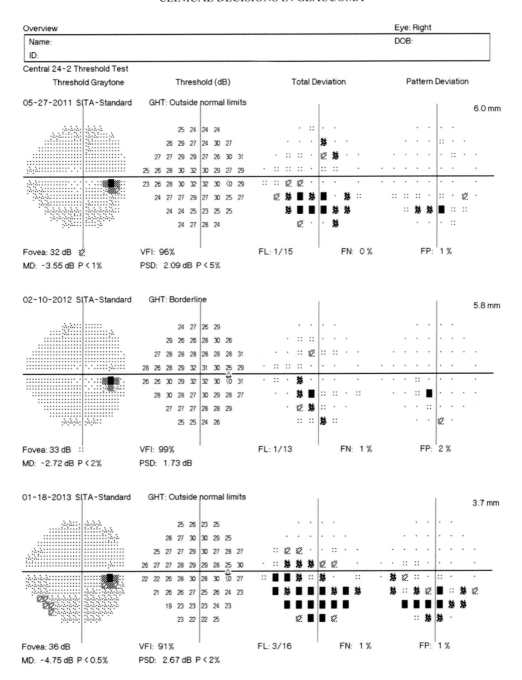

FIG 2-13. Overview. This condensed printout of a series of fields includes most of the information from the single-field analysis.

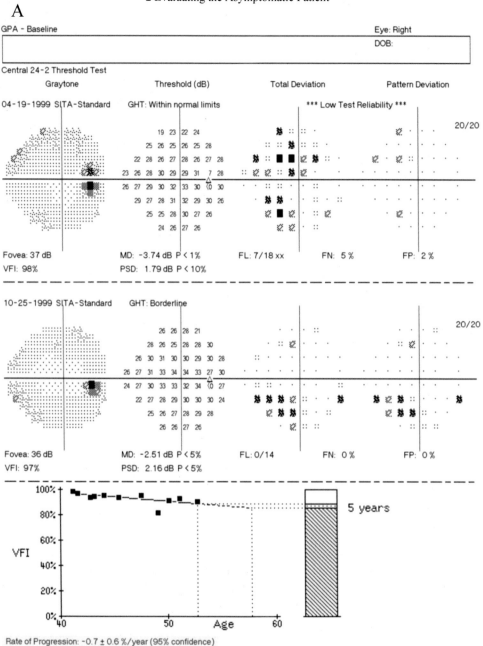

FIG 2-14. Guided Progression Analysis (GPA) Summary Report. **A.** (*this page*) GPA baseline and Visual Field Index (VFI) trend analysis. The patient's age is shown on the horizontal axis and VFI on the vertical axis. The rate of progression and likelihood that the changes occurred by chance are displayed below (*yellow highlight*). **B.** (*next page*) Glaucoma Change Probability Map (different patient). GPA alert shows "Possible Progression" if ≥ 3 test points deteriorated on <u>two</u> consecutive follow-up tests; "Likely Progression" (*yellow highlight*) if ≥ 3 test points deteriorated on <u>three</u> or more consecutive follow-up tests (open triangle = deterioration detected once, half-black triangle = deterioration detected on two consecutive exams, black triangle = deterioration detected on three consecutive exams). Detecting progression by visual field changes is discussed in Chapter 5.

B

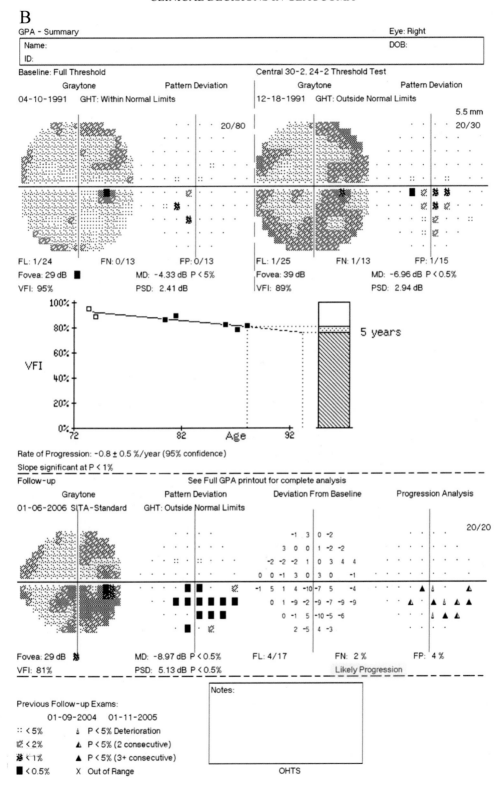

GPA - Summary

Eye: Right

| Name: | DOB: |
| ID: | |

Baseline: Full Threshold

Central 30-2, 24-2 Threshold Test

Graytone   Pattern Deviation

Graytone   Pattern Deviation

04-10-1991   GHT: Within Normal Limits

12-18-1991   GHT: Outside Normal Limits

5.5 mm

20/80

20/30

FL: 1/24   FN: 0/13   FP: 0/13

FL: 1/25   FN: 1/13   FP: 1/15

Fovea: 29 dB ■   MD: -4.33 dB P < 5%

Fovea: 39 dB   MD: -6.96 dB P < 0.5%

VFI: 95%   PSD: 2.41 dB

VFI: 89%   PSD: 2.94 dB

5 years

VFI

Age

Rate of Progression: -0.8 ± 0.5 %/year (95% confidence)

Slope significant at P < 1%

Follow-up   See Full GPA printout for complete analysis

Graytone   Pattern Deviation   Deviation From Baseline   Progression Analysis

01-06-2006 SITA-Standard   GHT: Outside Normal Limits

20/20

Fovea: 29 dB   MD: -8.97 dB P < 0.5%   FL: 4/17   FN: 2 %   FP: 4 %

VFI: 81%   PSD: 5.13 dB P < 0.5%   Likely Progression

Previous Follow-up Exams:

01-09-2004   01-11-2005

:: < 5%   ⌄ P < 5% Deterioration

� < 2%   ▲ P < 5% (2 consecutive)

⌫ < 1%   ▲ P < 5% (3+ consecutive)

■ < 0.5%   X Out of Range

Notes:

OHTS

Baseline Visual Field Examination

Future therapeutic decisions may depend on the relation between the baseline fields and subsequent fields; the more accurate the initial field baseline, the easier it is to determine on subsequent exams if a patient's condition is stable or changing. Patients with elevated pressure should have threshold tests. Although suprathreshold testing may be quite sensitive for identifying all but the most subtle defects, threshold testing permits much better comparison in the future.

We consider two fields to be the minimum baseline. For some individuals, more fields may be necessary. Fields vary from day to day, and multiple tests give a more accurate measurement than one test and provide a sense of the variability to be expected on different days in the patient. The time course for obtaining baseline fields is somewhat dependent on the patient's other findings. The more severe the damage, the more pressing the need to define the patient's position at the time of diagnosis and to proceed to therapy. We routinely obtain a 24-2 threshold test as the first field examination and perform a second 24-2 field examination within 1 or 2 months. If the first field is very depressed or constricted, we proceed as described on page 31. Depending on the similarity between the first two fields, additional early tests may be obtained to complete the baseline. Patients who require IOP-lowering may start treatment while their field baseline is being completed. This toilsome baseline effort improves the clinician's future ability to make accurate judgments. Henceforth, when the term *baseline* is used in relation to fields, we refer to at least two fields with the baseline determined as described below.

First two fields very similar, routine baseline. We consider the first two fields consistent and use the more reliable of the two as a baseline for future comparison if –

- The mean deviations (MD) differ by < 1.5dB regardless of defect severity, or
- The MD of both fields are -6 dB or worse and differ by < 2 dB.

First two fields vary, nonroutine baseline. The three common explanations for a marked difference between the first and second field are learning effect, marked true variability in the field, and poor patient reliability. Obtaining a third field helps to sort these and will, in most cases, complete the baseline studies.

Learning effect. Many people test better during perimetry after their first field. Some people improve a great deal, and in these individuals the baseline should exclude the first field. If the third field is similar to the second, use the second and third as a baseline. The GPA automatically analyzes a series of fields for reliability and learning effect and chooses two baseline exams. Occasionally a patient continues to improve with subsequent fields beyond the second (Figure 2-16). This makes establishment of a baseline difficult and frustrating, but the fields should be repeated fairly frequently until a consistent result is obtained. The severity of the other findings will guide the clinician in the timing of fields for the sake of a baseline – the more severe the disease, the more frequently the field should be tested until it stabilizes. Use the two or three most consistent fields as a baseline.

True variability or poor reliability. If the first three fields show random variation, attempt to determine whether the patient is reliable and the field is truly variable, or if the patient is not reliable. The assessment of reliability is reviewed on pages 42-49. If the patient seems to be reliable but the fields vary substantially, we generally rely on the Guided Progression Analysis program to select the best baseline fields.

If the fields vary widely and randomly and if it seems that the patient is unreliable, attempt to reeducate the patient as to how to perform perimetry. If this does not help, at some point it may be determined that threshold fields will not be useful. This is one instance when it is appropriate to try a suprathreshold field; if test length contributes to the patient's unreliability, suprathreshold testing may be better than nothing. If the patient simply cannot perform reliable field examinations, then he or she may be followed as described on pages 91-92 and 121-124.

First field very depressed or constricted –

Depression. The higher the threshold values and the more points seen, the better the basis to recognize changes. The standard 24-2 program uses a size III (4 mm^2) target. Retesting a very depressed field using a size V (64 mm^2) target may provide much more useful data (Figure 2-17). The STATPAC single-field analysis (to help determine if the field is normal or not) is not available for size V. However, the decision to use size V presumes that the field is clearly abnormal.

Marked constriction. If the majority of points seen on the 24-2 threshold test fall within the central 10 degrees, it is better to obtain a set of baseline 10-2 threshold tests. This program tests only the central 10 degrees using points separated by 2 degrees (Figures 2-15, 2-18). If the field is both depressed and constricted, a 10-2 program using a size V target may be useful (Figure 2-19).

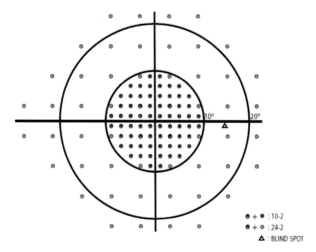

FIG 2-15. Test points on the 10-2 program. While the 24-2 tests (*blue dots*) point are separated by 6 degrees, 10-2 test points (*red dots*) are separated by only 2 degrees. Note that the 24-2 and 10-2 programs only overlap at one test point in each quadrant (*half-red, half-blue dots,* reprint from *Effective Perimetry, 4th Edition*, page 32, by A. Heijl et al, 2012, Dublin, CA: Carl Zeiss Meditec, Inc. Copyright 2012 by Carl Zeiss Meditec, Inc. Reprinted with permission).

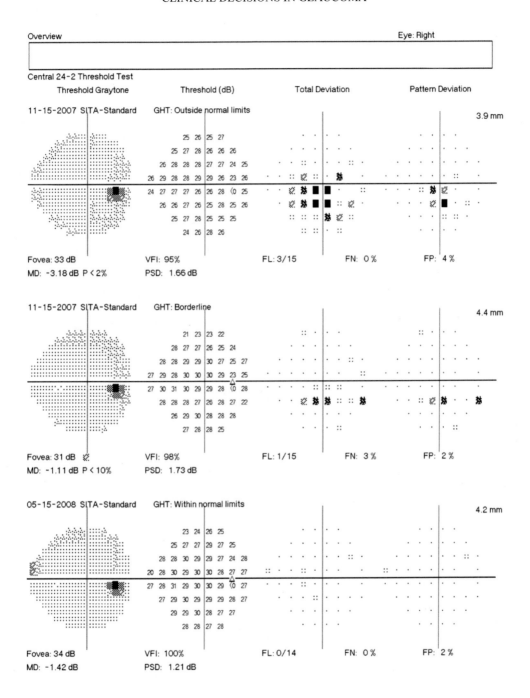

FIG 2-16. Learning effect. The first two fields were obtained on the same day. The first underestimated the patient's visual field and should not be part of the baseline for future comparison.

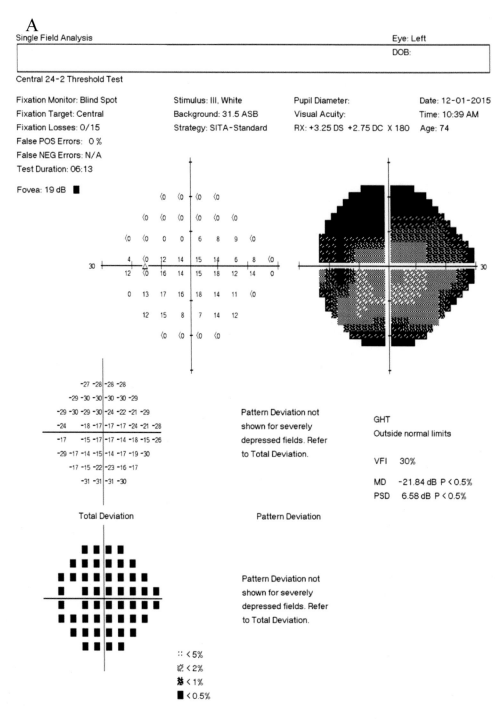

FIG 2-17. **A.** Depressed field, size III target. Threshold values are so depressed that progressive deterioration will be impossible to judge well. **B.** (*next page*) Depressed field, size V target. The defect depth plot highlights points that are particularly depressed relative to the overall field. The threshold sensitivities are high enough to follow. The total thresholds for each quadrant are displayed (*red circles*).

B

Three in One   Eye: Left

DOB:

Central 24-2 Threshold Test

Fixation Monitor: Blind Spot	Stimulus: V, White	Pupil Diameter:	Date: 12-01-2015
Fixation Target: Central	Background: 31.5 ASB	Visual Acuity:	Time: 10:52 AM
Fixation Losses: 0/17	Strategy: FASTPAC	RX: +3.25 DS +2.75 DC X 180	Age: 74
False POS Errors: 0/9			
False NEG Errors: 2/8			
Test Duration: 08:57			

Threshold Graytone

Fovea: 13 dB

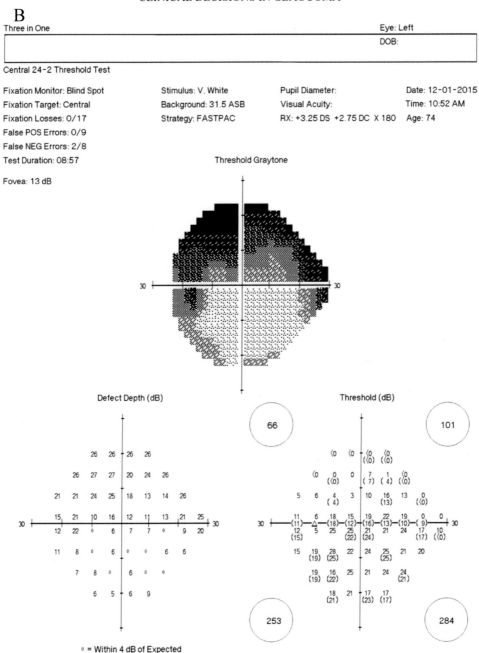

Defect Depth (dB)   Threshold (dB)

° = Within 4 dB of Expected

Central Reference: 30 dB xx

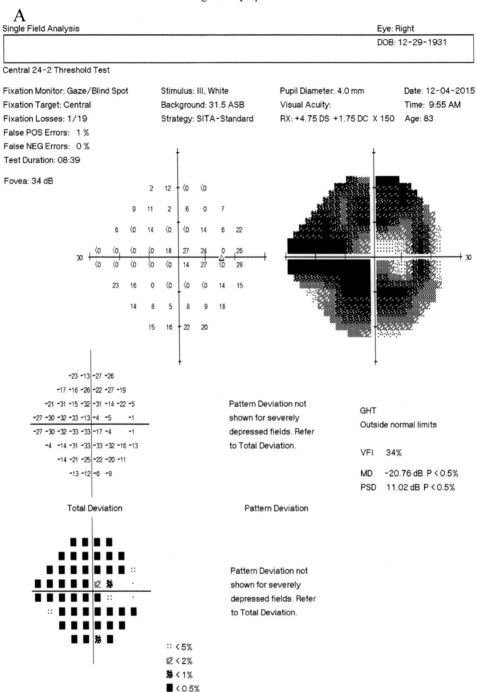

A

Single Field Analysis   Eye: Right

DOB: 12-29-1931

Central 24-2 Threshold Test

Fixation Monitor: Gaze/Blind Spot   Stimulus: III, White   Pupil Diameter: 4.0 mm   Date: 12-04-2015
Fixation Target: Central   Background: 31.5 ASB   Visual Acuity: Time: 9:55 AM
Fixation Losses: 1/19   Strategy: SITA-Standard   RX: +4.75 DS +1.75 DC X 150 Age: 83
False POS Errors: 1 %
False NEG Errors: 0 %
Test Duration: 08:39

Fovea: 34 dB

Total Deviation

Pattern Deviation not
shown for severely
depressed fields. Refer
to Total Deviation.

GHT
Outside normal limits

VFI   34%

MD   -20.76 dB P < 0.5%
PSD   11.02 dB P < 0.5%

Pattern Deviation

Pattern Deviation not
shown for severely
depressed fields. Refer
to Total Deviation.

:: < 5%
% < 2%
※ < 1%
■ < 0.5%

FIG 2-18. **A.** Constricted field. Only 5 points (excluding the fovea) are seen within 10 degrees of fixation. The patient was then tested with a 10-2 program. **B.** (*next page*) The 10-2 test on the same patient provides a larger number of test points to follow in the future. There is a slight worsening in reliability indices on retest, possibly related to patient fatigue. Multiple 10-2 fields can be printed in an overview.

B

Single Field Analysis

Eye: Right

)31

Central 10-2 Threshold Test

Fixation Monitor: Blind Spot
Fixation Target: Central
Fixation Losses: 6/19
False POS Errors: 6 %
False NEG Errors: 7 %
Test Duration: 09:26

Fovea: 34 dB

Stimulus: III, White
Background: 31.5 ASB
Strategy: SITA-Standard

Pupil Diameter: 4.0 mm
Visual Acuity:
RX: +4.75 DS +1.75 DC X 150

Date: 12-04-2015
Time: 10:19 AM
Age: 83

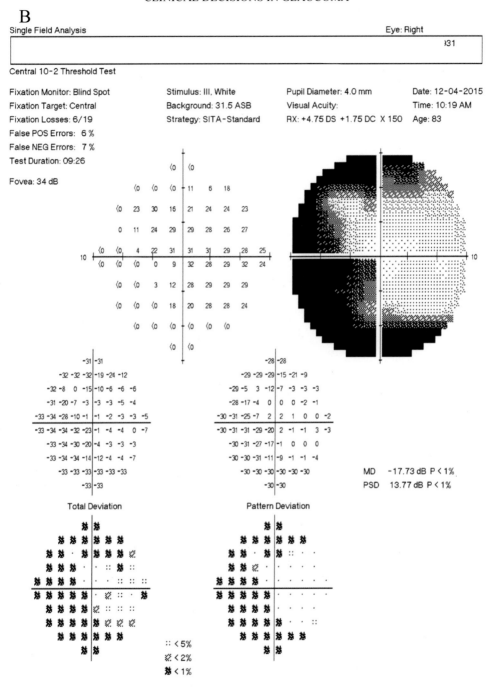

MD   -17.73 dB P < 1%
PSD   13.77 dB P < 1%

Total Deviation

Pattern Deviation

:: < 5%
∷ < 2%
≋ < 1%

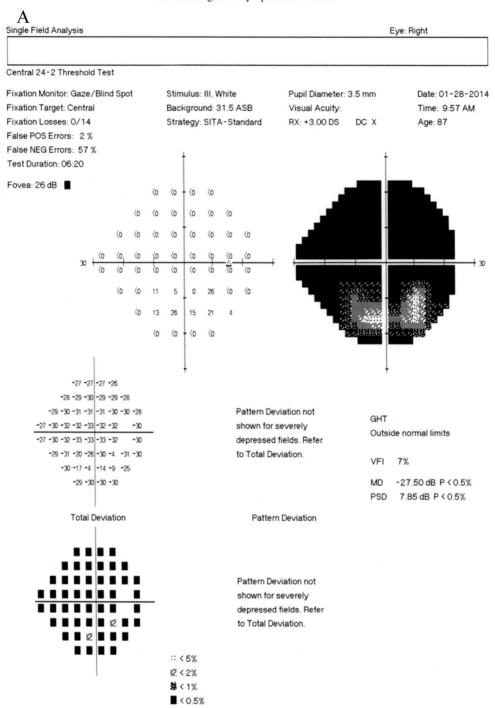

FIG 2-19. **A.** Depressed and constricted field. 24-2 program with size III (4 mm²) target. The size III target was seen in only a few points. **B.** (*next page*) 10-2 program with size V (64 mm²) target on the same patient provides a larger number of test points to follow in the future.

B

Three in One   Eye: Right

Central 10-2 Threshold Test

Fixation Monitor: Gaze/Blind Spot	Stimulus: V, White	Pupil Diameter: 3.6 mm	Date: 01-28-2014
Fixation Target: Central	Background: 31.5 ASB	Visual Acuity:	Time: 5:11 PM
Fixation Losses: 3/17	Strategy: FASTPAC	RX: +3.50 DS DC X	Age: 87
False POS Errors: 2/12			
False NEG Errors: 0/10			
Test Duration: 10:54			

Fovea: 19 dB

Threshold Graytone

Defect Depth (dB)

```
                    26  26
            25  29  28 | 26  23  25
        28  27  26  20 | 27  20  26  22
        24  24  16  20 | 13  12  23  21
   18  16  17  17  12  |  5   6  10  11  17
10 +----------------------------------------- 10
    7   6   7   ◦   8   ◦   ◦   ◦   ◦   ◦
    ◦   7   ◦   ◦ | 12  15  13  11
    ◦   ◦  10   ◦ | 13  16  11  11
         8   8  14 | 14  14  13
                 8 | 11
```

Threshold (dB)

```
115                                              176
                        2 | 2
              3    0    2 | 3    6    3
                 ( 0) ( 0)|
         0    0    3    9 | 1   13    4    6
            ( 3) ( 3)     |( 4) ( 4) ( 1)
              8    6   13  9 | 16   22    7    6
            ( 2) ( 3) (13)   |     (13) ( 4) ( 9)
        10   11   12   12 | 18   25   25   19   18   11
       (14)      (18)-(25)-(22)                (11)+ 10
10 +-----------------------------------------------+ 10
        20   20   22   25 | 22   25   25   25   29   23
       (23) (26)         |(28) (25) (31) (26) (29)
        27   22   28   25 | 19   16   19   18
                 (25)     +(16) (13) (13)
        24   25   19   25 | 16   10   19   17
            (25) (19)     |     (16) (16)
             20   21   15 | 15   15   15
                    (15)  |
383              20 | 17                          324
```

◦ = Within 4 dB of Expected
Central Reference: 30 dB xx

Visual Field Interpretation

The interpretation of a visual field involves three steps – recognition of artifact, determination of reliability, and assessment for evidence of damage.

Artifact. Two common field artifacts are those caused by the upper lid and the lens rim. The lid artifact is always superior and thus easier to recognize. A lens rim artifact appears if a corrective lens is either too far from the eye or is not centered. In either case the rim of the lens projects into the test area. Lens rim artifacts are usually sharply demarcated absolute defects with sensitivity of 0 dB (Figure 2-20 A and B).

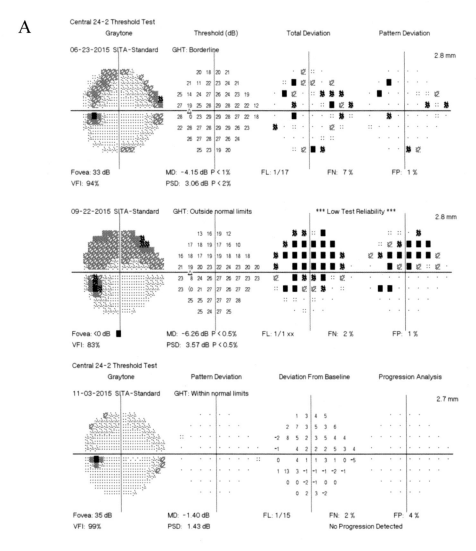

FIG 2-20. Artifacts in visual field examination. **A.** *(this page)* Lid artifact. The first two fields showed worsening superior defects. On the most recent visual field, the upper lid was taped up and the field returned to normal. **B.** *(next page)* Lens rim artifact with sharply demarcated absolute defects (*yellow highlights*).

B

Central 24-2 Threshold Test

Fixation Monitor: Blind Spot	Stimulus: V, White	Pupil Diameter:
Fixation Target: Central	Background: 31.5 ASB	Visual Acuity:
Fixation Losses: 2/17	Strategy: FASTPAC	RX: +16.75 DS +3.25 DC X 55
False POS Errors: 0/10		
False NEG Errors: 0/8		
Test Duration: 09:28		

Date: 12-10-2015
Time: 10:30 AM
Age: 72

Fovea: 18 dB

Threshold Graytone

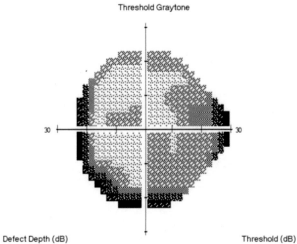

Defect Depth (dB)

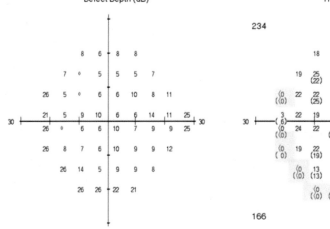

Threshold (dB)

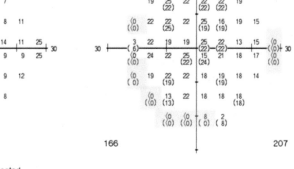

◦ = Within 4 dB of Expected
Central Reference: 30 dB xx

Reliability. Reliability estimates depend on three main signs (in descending order of importance): false-positive rate, false-negative rate, and fixation loss rate. The clinician should determine the reliability of each field.

False positives. If the patient responds any time that a stimulus could not have been seen, e.g. before stimulus presentation, the machine records a false-positive response. False positives are caused neither by eye pathology nor testing artifact (except in the rare patient with photopsia). They randomly change the contour of the hill of vision and distort the true map of retinal sensitivities. They are almost always a marker of real unreliability. The perimeter will signal low reliability if the false-positive rate is $\geq 33\%$ (Figure 2-21), but we regard fields with a $\geq 5\%$ false-positive rate as probably unreliable. We reject visual fields with $\geq 10\%$ false positives. Reliable fields can usually be obtained by educating the patient to be reasonably certain of seeing the stimulus, not to respond in haste (no need to respond while the stimulus is still on), and to expect stimuli that he or she cannot see. In such cases, the baseline examinations should be obtained after the education (Figure 2-22). If educating a patient does not result in a more reliable field, then fields may simply not be helpful in that patient.

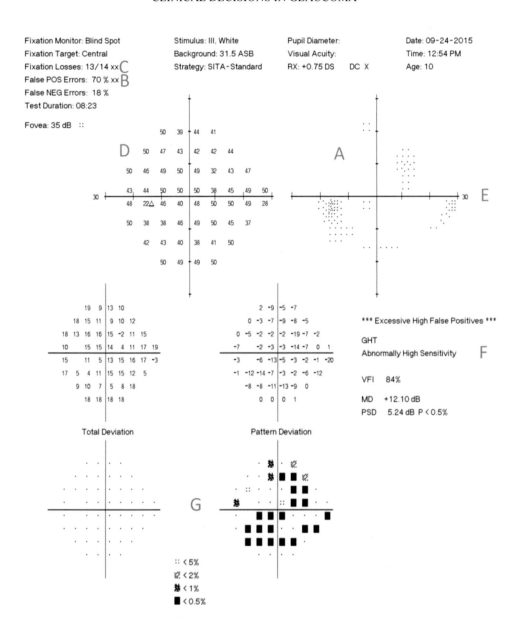

Fixation Monitor: Blind Spot
Fixation Target: Central
Fixation Losses: 13/14 xx C
False POS Errors: 70 % xx B
False NEG Errors: 18 %
Test Duration: 08:23

Fovea: 35 dB ::

Stimulus: III, White
Background: 31.5 ASB
Strategy: SITA-Standard

Pupil Diameter:
Visual Acuity:
RX: +0.75 DS   DC X

Date: 09-24-2015
Time: 12:54 PM
Age: 10

*** Excessive High False Positives ***

GHT
Abnormally High Sensitivity

VFI   84%

MD   +12.10 dB
PSD   5.24 dB P < 0.5%

Total Deviation

Pattern Deviation

:: < 5%
⚏ < 2%
⚎ < 1%
■ < 0.5%

FIG 2-21. High false-positive rate. There are seven findings related to an excessively high false-positive rate. **A.** White scotoma on gray scale. **B.** High false positives. **C.** High fixation loss rate. The field analyzer records any response to a stimulus projected onto the physiologic blind spot as a fixation loss, which occurs with increased frequency in an examination with a high false-positive rate. **D.** Supra-normal sensitivities (higher than foveal sensitivity, which is 35 dB in this case). **E.** Loss of the physiologic blind spot. **F.** The Glaucoma Hemifield Test message "Abnormally High Sensitivity," which appears when the overall sensitivity in the best part of the field is higher than that found in 99.5% of the population. **G.** "Reverse cataract" pattern in which generalized depression occurs on the pattern deviation rather than total deviation.

A

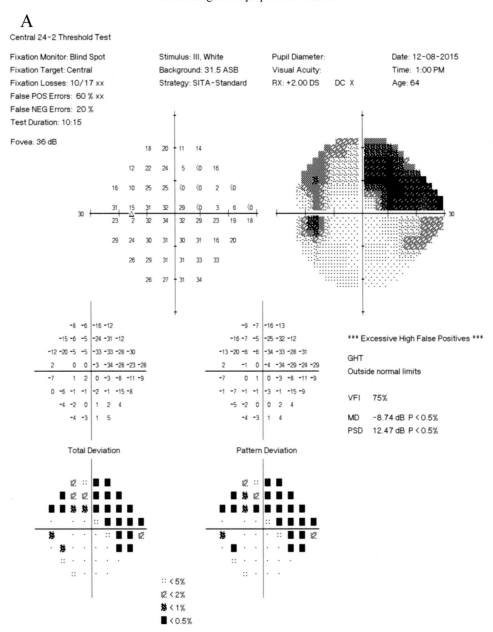

FIG 2-22. High false-positive rate. **A.** (*this page*) The 24-2 field is so abnormal that the clinician might be tempted to entirely abandon perimetry. However, the patient was educated in how to respond, and the test pattern was switched to 10-2. **B.** (*next page*) Visual field by the same patient with markedly improved reliability indices.

B

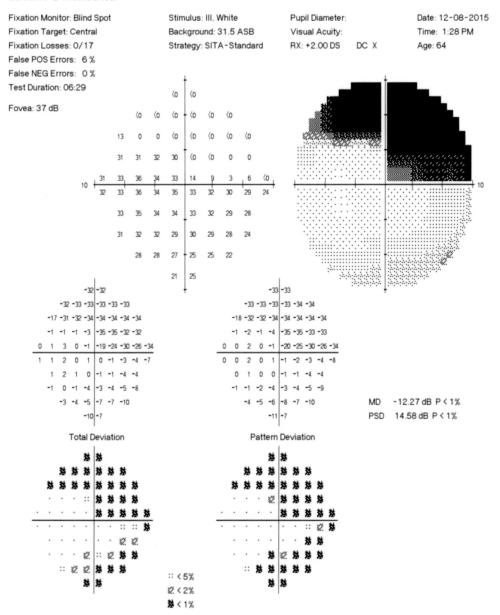

Central 10-2 Threshold Test

Fixation Monitor: Blind Spot
Fixation Target: Central
Fixation Losses: 0/17
False POS Errors: 6 %
False NEG Errors: 0 %
Test Duration: 06:29

Fovea: 37 dB

Stimulus: III, White
Background: 31.5 ASB
Strategy: SITA-Standard

Pupil Diameter:
Visual Acuity:
RX: +2.00 DS   DC X

Date: 12-08-2015
Time: 1:28 PM
Age: 64

MD   -12.27 dB P < 1%
PSD   14.58 dB P < 1%

Total Deviation

Pattern Deviation

:: < 5%
⌀ < 2%
▓ < 1%

False negatives. False-negative responses – a failure to respond to a stimulus 9 dB brighter than one previously seen at the same location – do not necessarily indicate unreliable fields. Inconsistent responses characterize regions of depressed sensitivity, and a brighter stimulus may truly not be visible on second presentation (Figure 2-23). Conversely, a tired patient may fail to respond to a stimulus that was previously visible to him or her. In this situation the field test is unreliable. Interpret fields with many false-negative responses in light of the entire clinical picture.

One characteristic field defect seen in people with high false-negative rates related to fatigue is the "cloverleaf" field in which the patient responds to the early test points but then fails to respond to subsequent stimuli. A variant of this field is the apparently constricted field, a "pseudocentral island," in which the patient failed to respond to the points tested last which were, because of the test logic, the peripheral points (Figure 2-24).

Fixation losses. Not all fixation losses represent true loss of fixation. The Humphrey perimeter monitors fixation by either the Heijl-Krakau method or by use of a videographic monitoring device. [11] In the Heijl-Krakau method, the perimeter first quickly locates the blind spot and then projects an occasional maximum stimulus into it. If the patient responds to the stimulus, a shift in the blind spot and fixation has occurred, and the machine records a fixation loss. A high number of fixation losses may thus indicate that the center of the blind spot was slightly mislocated. A high false-positive rate will give a high fixation loss rate as well (Figure 2-21). The gaze tracker uses videographic image analysis to locate and track the movement of the center of the pupil and the reflection of a lighted target off of the corneal surface and is precise to approximately ± 1°. During each stimulus presentation, a deviated gaze is shown as an upward-extending line (the length is proportional to the amount of deviation, up to 10°). An inability to gauge gaze direction (e.g. pupil and/or corneal reflex blocked during a blink) is shown as a downward-extending line in the gaze tracking record (located at the bottom of the Single Field Analysis printout, Figure 2-12J).

If the false-positive and false-negative rates are low, we discount a high fixation loss rate. We also discount it if the two baseline fields are very similar (Figure 2-25).

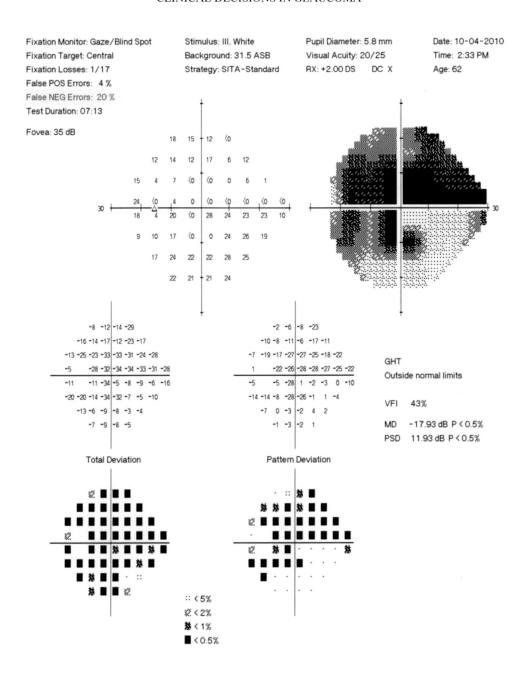

Fixation Monitor: Gaze/Blind Spot
Fixation Target: Central
Fixation Losses: 1/17
False POS Errors: 4 %
False NEG Errors: 20 %
Test Duration: 07:13

Fovea: 35 dB

Stimulus: III, White
Background: 31.5 ASB
Strategy: SITA-Standard

Pupil Diameter: 5.8 mm
Visual Acuity: 20/25
RX: +2.00 DS   DC X

Date: 10-04-2010
Time: 2:33 PM
Age: 62

GHT
Outside normal limits

VFI   43%

MD   −17.93 dB P < 0.5%
PSD   11.93 dB P < 0.5%

Total Deviation

Pattern Deviation

:: < 5%
⬚ < 2%
❋ < 1%
■ < 0.5%

FIG 2-23. High false-negative rate in a severely damaged field. In this widely damaged field, the false-negative rate (*yellow highlight*) is probably related to true variability. There are very few fixation losses and false positives.

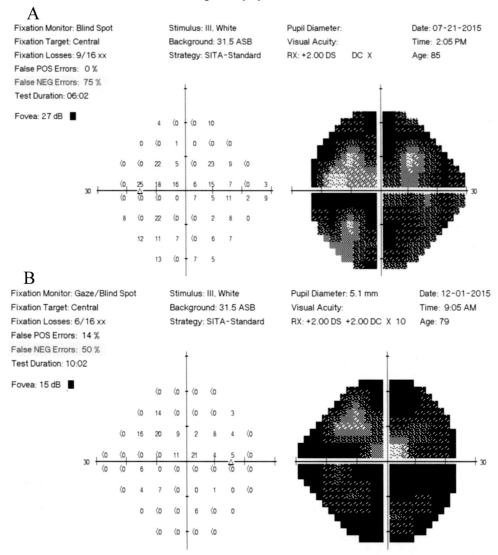

A

Fixation Monitor: Blind Spot
Fixation Target: Central
Fixation Losses: 9/16 xx
False POS Errors: 0 %
False NEG Errors: 75 %
Test Duration: 06:02

Fovea: 27 dB

Stimulus: III, White
Background: 31.5 ASB
Strategy: SITA-Standard

Pupil Diameter:
Visual Acuity:
RX: +2.00 DS   DC X

Date: 07-21-2015
Time: 2:05 PM
Age: 85

B

Fixation Monitor: Gaze/Blind Spot
Fixation Target: Central
Fixation Losses: 6/16 xx
False POS Errors: 14 %
False NEG Errors: 50 %
Test Duration: 10:02

Fovea: 15 dB

Stimulus: III, White
Background: 31.5 ASB
Strategy: SITA-Standard

Pupil Diameter: 5.1 mm
Visual Acuity:
RX: +2.00 DS +2.00 DC X 10

Date: 12-01-2015
Time: 9:05 AM
Age: 79

FIG 2-24. High false-negative rate due to fatigue. **A.** Cloverleaf field (see text). **B.** Pseudocentral island related to rapid fatigue in a normal individual.

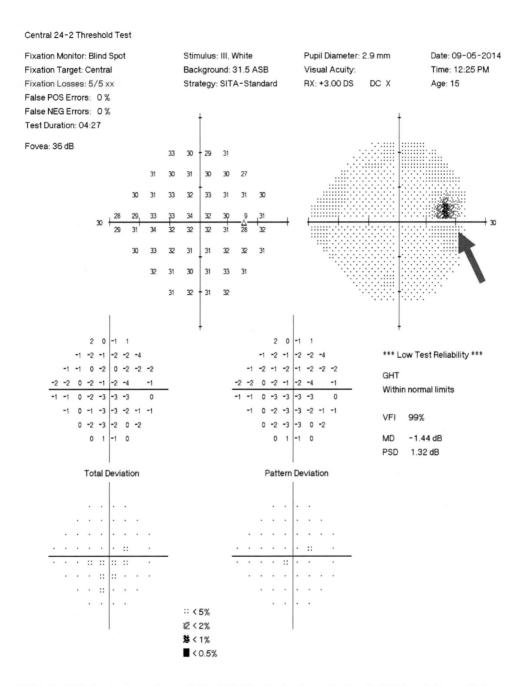

Central 24-2 Threshold Test

Fixation Monitor: Blind Spot	Stimulus: III, White	Pupil Diameter: 2.9 mm	Date: 09-05-2014
Fixation Target: Central	Background: 31.5 ASB	Visual Acuity:	Time: 12:25 PM
Fixation Losses: 5/5 xx	Strategy: SITA-Standard	RX: +3.00 DS DC X	Age: 15

False POS Errors: 0 %
False NEG Errors: 0 %
Test Duration: 04:27

Fovea: 36 dB

*** Low Test Reliability ***

GHT
Within normal limits

VFI   99%

MD   -1.44 dB
PSD   1.32 dB

Total Deviation

Pattern Deviation

:: < 5%
▨ < 2%
▩ < 1%
■ < 0.5%

FIG 2-25. High fixation losses in a reliable field. The fixation losses (*yellow highlight*) probably result from mislocation of the center of the blind spot (*arrow*). Other reliability parameters are adequate.

Normality and Abnormality

Despite the impossibility (and relative therapeutic unimportance) of classifying equivocal fields as normal or abnormal, both doctors and patients want to know if a field shows acquired damage. Obvious defects pose no diagnostic dilemmas. However, the earliest defects of glaucoma are often equivocal. A very good determinant of the presence of glaucomatous damage on a single field is the Glaucoma Hemifield Test (GHT), which compares corresponding areas in the superior and inferior hemifields (Figures 2-26 and 2-27). This analysis relates only to glaucoma, and it always should be interpreted in light of the rest of the clinical picture. It does not, for example, analyze temporal nerve fiber bundle defects or vertical hemianopias (Figure 2-28).

In the absence of other cause for field abnormality and in the presence of a suspicion of glaucoma, a hemifield test outside normal limits on both (or on a minimum of two) baseline field examinations strongly suggests that the patient has glaucoma. Two other reliable indicators of acquired damage are (1) a cluster of three or more points in a location typical for glaucoma, all of which are depressed on the pattern deviation plot at a p < 5% level and one of which is depressed at a p < 1 % level (Figures 2-29 and 2-30), and (2) a pattern standard deviation that occurs in less than 5% of normal fields (Figures 2-31, see HAP2 criteria part I, page 53). In all cases, the visual fields should be reliable and reproducible.

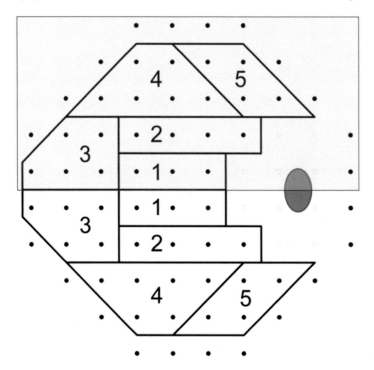

FIG 2-26. Glaucoma hemifield test. The five numbered zones in the upper hemifield (*red box*) are compared to corresponding zones in the lower hemifield. The program also compares the overall height of the hill of vision to age-adjusted normal.

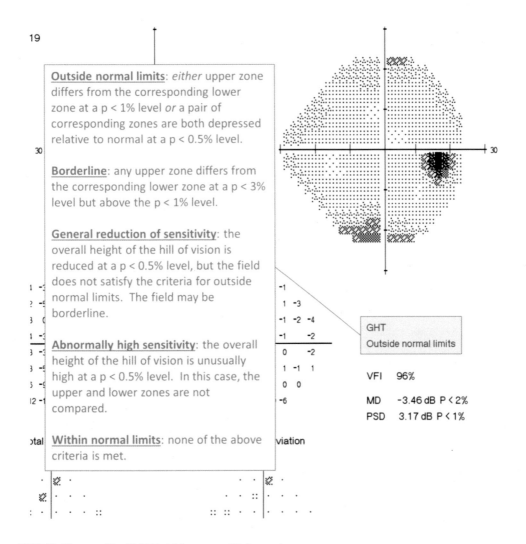

19

Outside normal limits: *either* upper zone differs from the corresponding lower zone at a p < 1% level *or* a pair of corresponding zones are both depressed relative to normal at a p < 0.5% level.

Borderline: any upper zone differs from the corresponding lower zone at a p < 3% level but above the p < 1% level.

General reduction of sensitivity: the overall height of the hill of vision is reduced at a p < 0.5% level, but the field does not satisfy the criteria for outside normal limits. The field may be borderline.

Abnormally high sensitivity: the overall height of the hill of vision is unusually high at a p < 0.5% level. In this case, the upper and lower zones are not compared.

Within normal limits: none of the above criteria is met.

GHT
Outside normal limits

VFI   96%

MD   -3.46 dB P < 2%
PSD   3.17 dB P < 1%

FIG 2-27. Glaucoma Hemifield Test. Messages and their meanings.

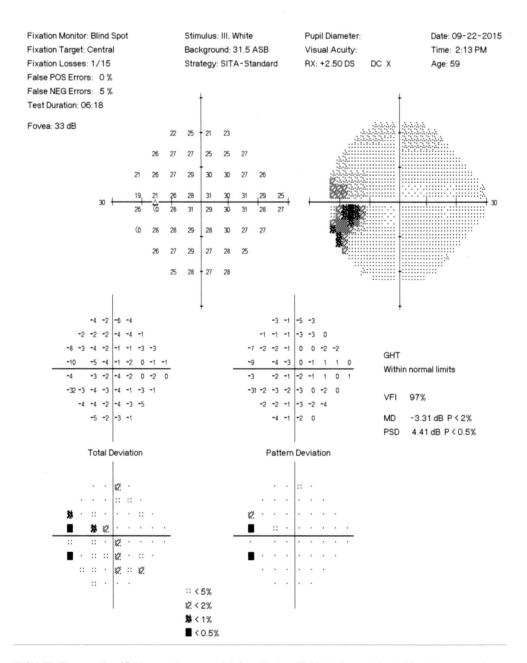

Fixation Monitor: Blind Spot
Fixation Target: Central
Fixation Losses: 1/15
False POS Errors: 0 %
False NEG Errors: 5 %
Test Duration: 06:18

Fovea: 33 dB

Stimulus: III, White
Background: 31.5 ASB
Strategy: SITA-Standard

Pupil Diameter:
Visual Acuity:
RX: +2.50 DS   DC X

Date: 09-22-2015
Time: 2:13 PM
Age: 59

GHT
Within normal limits

VFI   97%

MD   -3.31 dB P < 2%
PSD   4.41 dB P < 0.5%

Total Deviation

Pattern Deviation

:: < 5%
⊠ < 2%
⊠ < 1%
■ < 0.5%

FIG 2-28. Glaucoma hemifield test and a temporal defect. The hemifield test does not deal with points temporal to the disc. This deep defect did not affect the hemifield results.

Since published in the first edition of this book in 1993, the Hodapp-Anderson-Parrish (HAP) criteria for visual field interpretation have been utilized in multiple large clinical studies.[12-19] They describe the minimal criteria for diagnosing acquired glaucomatous damage, offer a reasonable classification of defects, and outline criteria to determine field progression. In the current edition, we have updated the HAP criteria (HAP2) to reflect several important changes since the first publication. These include:

- The popularization of the 24-2 visual field in place of the 30-2 visual field
- The use of pattern standard deviation (PSD) instead of corrected pattern standard deviation (CPSD)
- The development of the Visual Field Index (VFI)
- The use of the Guided Progression Analysis (GPA)

VFI represents the weighted summary of a patient's visual field status, and is expressed as a percentage of the normal, age-corrected sensitivity. A normal visual field has a VFI of 100%. PSD summarizes the extent of localized loss and is not affected by generalized depression. PSD is low in normal fields, in uniformly depressed fields, and in totally extinguished fields. It is highest in moderate to severe localized loss. GPA is reviewed on pages 28-29.

HAP2 criteria for visual field interpretation. The HAP2 criteria consist of three parts:

- Part I – Minimal criteria for diagnosing acquired glaucomatous damage (see box below)
- Part II – Classification of glaucomatous visual field defects (Chapter 3)
- Part III – Criteria for visual field progression (Chapter 5)

The HAP2 criteria assume that the visual fields to which they are applied are reasonably reliable and reproducible, and that glaucoma is the cause of the visual field defects.

HAP2 Criteria, Part I
Minimum Criteria for Diagnosing Acquired Glaucomatous Damage in a 24-2 Examination

Any of the following must be reproducible on two consecutive fields –

- A Glaucoma Hemifield Test "Outside normal limits."
- A cluster of three or more points in a location typical for glaucoma, all of which are depressed on the pattern deviation plot at a $p < 5\%$ level and one of which is depressed at a $p < 1\%$ level.
- A pattern standard deviation that occurs in less than 5% of normal fields.

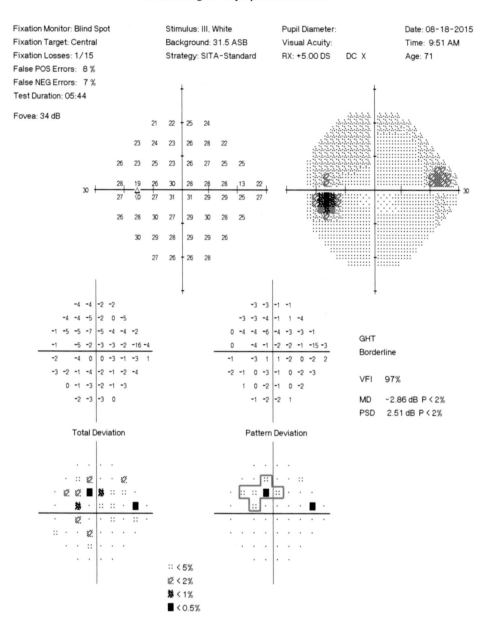

Fixation Monitor: Blind Spot
Fixation Target: Central
Fixation Losses: 1/15
False POS Errors: 8 %
False NEG Errors: 7 %
Test Duration: 05:44

Fovea: 34 dB

Stimulus: III, White
Background: 31.5 ASB
Strategy: SITA-Standard

Pupil Diameter:
Visual Acuity:
RX: +5.00 DS   DC X

Date: 08-18-2015
Time: 9:51 AM
Age: 71

GHT
Borderline

VFI   97%

MD   -2.86 dB P < 2%
PSD   2.51 dB P < 2%

Total Deviation

Pattern Deviation

:: < 5%
< 2%
< 1%
■ < 0.5%

FIG 2-29. Minimal pattern deviation criteria for acquired abnormality. At least three (here six, *outlined*) clustered points each depressed at a 5% level and one at least at a 1% (here 0.5%) level. This defect was confirmed on repeat testing.

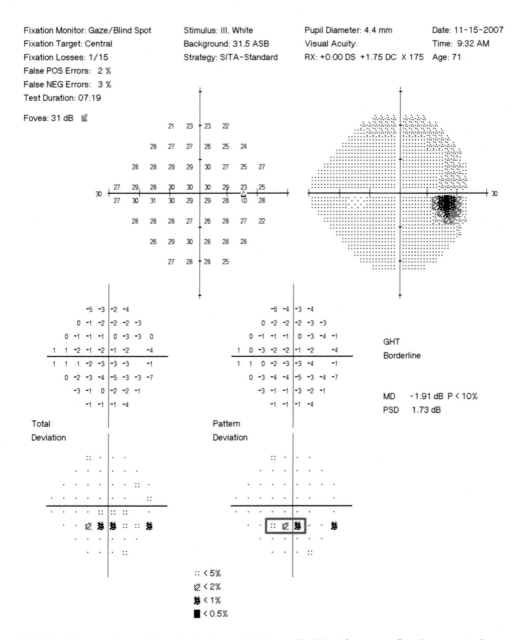

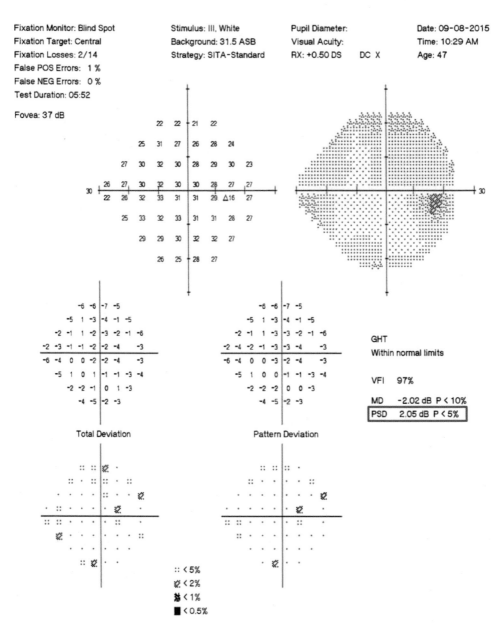

Fixation Monitor: Blind Spot
Fixation Target: Central
Fixation Losses: 2/14
False POS Errors: 1 %
False NEG Errors: 0 %
Test Duration: 05:52

Fovea: 37 dB

Stimulus: III, White
Background: 31.5 ASB
Strategy: SITA-Standard

Pupil Diameter:
Visual Acuity:
RX: +0.50 DS   DC X

Date: 09-08-2015
Time: 10:29 AM
Age: 47

GHT
Within normal limits

VFI   97%

MD   -2.02 dB P < 10%
PSD   2.05 dB P < 5%

Total Deviation

Pattern Deviation

:: < 5%
⍉ < 2%
⊗ < 1%
■ < 0.5%

FIG 2-31. Minimum pattern standard deviation (PSD) criterion for acquired damage. PSD < 5% is the sole finding in this visual field. Note that there are no clusters of three or more points all of which are depressed on the pattern deviation plot at a p < 5% level and one of which is depressed at a p < 1 % level, and the Glaucoma Hemifield Test is "Within normal limits." The finding was confirmed on repeat testing. This patient presented with elevated intraocular pressures and has increased cupping.

References

1. Allingham RR, Damji K, Freedman S Moroi S, Shafranov G. Eds. Shields' Textbook of Glaucoma. Lippincott Williams & Wilkins, Philadelphia, PA, USA. 2005.

2. Groh MJ, Küchle M. Idiopathic episcleral venous stasis with secondary open angle glaucoma (Radius-Maumenee syndrome)]. Klinische Monatsblätter für Augenheilkunde. 1997 Aug;211(2):131-2.

3. Swanson MW. The 97.5th and 99.5th percentile of vertical cup disc ratio in the United States. Optometry & Vision Science. 2011 Jan;88(1):86-92.

4. Drance SM. Disc hemorrhages in the glaucomas. Survey of Ophthalmology. 1989 Mar-Apr;33(5):331-7.

5. Liu Y, Simavli H, Que CJ, Rizzo JL, Tsikata E, Maurer R, Chen TC. Patient characteristics associated with artifacts in Spectralis optical coherence tomography imaging of the retinal nerve fiber layer in glaucoma. American Journal of Ophthalmology. 2015 Mar;159(3):565-76.

6. Kim NR, Lee H, Lee ES, Kim JH, Hong S, Je Seong G, Kim CY. Influence of cataract on time domain and spectral domain optical coherence tomography retinal nerve fiber layer measurements. Journal of Glaucoma. 2012 Feb;21(2):116-22.

7. Russell DJ, Fallah S, Loer CJ, Riffenburgh RH. A comprehensive model for correcting RNFL readings of varying signal strengths in cirrus optical coherence tomography. Investigative Ophthalmology & Visual Science. 2014 Oct 16;55(11):7297-302.

8. Chang RT, Knight OJ, Feuer WJ, Budenz DL. Sensitivity and specificity of time-domain versus spectral-domain optical coherence tomography in diagnosing early to moderate glaucoma. Ophthalmology. 2009 Dec;116(12):2294-9.

9. Asrani S, Essaid L, Alder BD, Santiago-Turla C. Artifacts in spectral-domain optical coherence tomography measurements in glaucoma. JAMA Ophthalmology. 2014 Apr 1;132(4):396-402.

10. El-Dairi M, Holgado S, Asrani S, Freedman SF. Optical coherence tomography (OCT) measurements in black and white children with large cup-to-disc ratios. Experimental Eye Research. 2011 Sep;93(3):299-307.

11. Heijl A, Patella VM, Bengtsson B. The Field Analyzer Primer, Fourth Edition: Effective Perimetry. Dublin, California: Carl Zeiss Meditec, Inc. 2012. Print.

12. Asakawa K, Kato S, Shoji N, Morita T, Shimizu K. Evaluation of optic nerve head using a newly developed stereo retinal imaging technique by glaucoma specialist and non-expert-

certified orthoptist. Journal of Glaucoma. 2013 Dec;22(9):698-706.

13. Budenz DL, Rhee P, Feuer WJ, McSoley J, Johnson CA, Anderson DR. Comparison of glaucomatous visual field defects using standard full threshold and Swedish interactive threshold algorithms. Archives of Ophthalmology. 2002 Sep;120(9):1136-41.

14. Gracitelli CP, Duque-Chica GL, Moura AL, Nagy BV, de Melo GR, Roizenblatt M, Borba PD, Teixeira SH, Ventura DF, Paranhos A Jr. A positive association between intrinsically photosensitive retinal ganglion cells and retinal nerve fiber layer thinning in glaucoma. Investigative Ophthalmology & Visual Science. 2014 Nov 18;55(12):7997-8005.

15. Labiris G, Katsanos A, Fanariotis M, Zacharaki F, Chatzoulis D, Kozobolis VP. Vision-specific quality of life in Greek glaucoma patients. Journal of Glaucoma. 2010 Jan;19(1):39-43.

16. Lakshmanan Y, George RJ. Stereoacuity in mild, moderate and severe glaucoma. Ophthalmic Physiological Optics. 2013 Mar;33(2):172-8.

17. Lee PP, Walt JG, Doyle JJ, Kotak SV, Evans SJ, Budenz DL, Chen PP, Coleman AL, Feldman RM, Jampel HD, Katz LJ, Mills RP, Myers JS, Noecker RJ, Piltz-Seymour JR, Ritch RR, Schacknow PN, Serle JB, Trick GL. A multicenter, retrospective pilot study of resource use and costs associated with severity of disease in glaucoma. Archives of Ophthalmology. 2006 Jan;124(1):12-9.

18. Li T, Liu Z, Li J, Liu Z, Tang Z, Xie X, Yang D, Wang N, Tian J, Xian J. Altered amplitude of low-frequency fluctuation in primary open angle glaucoma: a resting-state FMRI study. Investigative Ophthalmology & Visual Science. 2014 Dec 18;56(1):322-9.

19. Mills RP, Budenz DL, Lee PP, Noecker RJ, Walt JG, Siegartel LR, Evans SJ, Doyle JJ. Categorizing the stage of glaucoma from pre-diagnosis to end-stage disease. American Journal of Ophthalmology. 2006 Jan;141(1):24-30.

3 DIAGNOSING GLAUCOMA

At the conclusion of the ***initial*** evaluation, the asymptomatic patient can be placed in one of the following categories based on the intraocular pressure (IOP), slit lamp examination, gonioscopy, optic disc and retinal nerve fiber layer (RNFL) imaging, and visual field findings (Chart 3-1) –

1. Glaucoma suspect due to ocular hypertension (primary or secondary; RNFL *or* visual field abnormalities may be present),
2. Glaucoma suspect due to an abnormal disc and/or visual field finding with low or normal IOP that makes a glaucoma diagnosis uncertain,
3. Glaucoma suspect due to an abnormal angle appearance only,
4. Manifest glaucoma (glaucomatous damage is present based on functional *and* structural examinations in an eye with elevated IOP).

On *subsequent* evaluation, some glaucoma suspects may convert to manifest glaucoma by demonstrating changes consistent with progressive, acquired damage, while others, especially those treated presumptively after the initial evaluation, may remain suspects.

Patient categories	IOP > 21 mmHg	Circumpapillary OCT-RNFL findings			Visual field findings
		Abnormal thickness, normal contour	Normal thickness, abnormal contour	Abnormal thickness/contour	Visual field abnormal
		One or more of the above			
Glaucoma suspect: Ocular hypertension	+		-		-
			+		-
			-		+
Glaucoma suspect: Abnormal disc and/or visual field	-		+		+
			+		-
			-		+
Glaucoma suspect: Abnormal angle	-		-		-
Manifest glaucoma	+		+		+

CHART 3-1. Patient categories after ***initial*** glaucoma evaluation. The table does not suggest that an elevated pressure is a diagnostic requirement for manifest glaucoma. Patients who present with optic disc and/or visual field findings suggestive of glaucoma in the absence of elevated pressure during the ***initial*** evaluation are categorized as glaucoma suspects until nonglaucomatous etiologies have been ruled out (see text). Key – IOP (intraocular pressure), OCT-RNFL (optical coherence tomography retinal nerve fiber layer analysis).

Glaucoma Diagnosis Based on the Initial Evaluation

We diagnose glaucoma in an adult when the patient's examination and course show the presence of a chronic, progressive optic neuropathy characterized by –

1. Optic disc cupping, accompanied by thinning or notching of the neuroretinal rim, with corresponding visual field defects, or
2. Ongoing changes in the optic nerve consistent with glaucomatous damage as documented by serial stereoscopic disc photographs or comparable imaging modalities, even if visual field defects are absent or cannot be demonstrated.

During the *initial* evaluation, a patient is diagnosed with glaucoma if he or she presents with structural <u>and</u> functional findings of glaucoma in the context of elevated IOP. Unless the patient brings with him/her the results of prior high-quality, diagnostic studies, it is impossible to infer an active, ongoing pathologic process in the optic disc based on a solitary examination. However, while elevated IOP does not define glaucoma, when *both* structural and functional abnormalities consistent with optic nerve damage are present in the context of elevated IOP, we presume that the damage is glaucomatous and ongoing, even though the "chronic" and "progressive" nature of the disease has not yet been demonstrated. On the other hand, when these findings present without IOP elevation, there are several possibilities:

1. The findings are normal physiologic variants and/or testing artifacts mimicking acquired damage;
2. The damage is real but not glaucomatous in nature (e.g. compressive lesions);
3. The damage is real and glaucomatous, but occurred during prior episode(s) of IOP elevation and is no longer ongoing;
4. The damage is real, glaucomatous and ongoing at an IOP that is within the statistically normal range.

When a patient presents with elevated IOP and either a visual field abnormality *or* an abnormal RNFL, but not both, the absence of structural/functional correlation makes the glaucoma diagnosis uncertain. We categorize these patients as glaucoma suspects after the initial evaluation until testing artifacts and nonglaucomatous pathologies have been ruled out during subsequent evaluations. The topic of whether to initiate presumptive treatment in a glaucoma suspect is explored in subsequent chapters.

Glaucoma Diagnosis during the Subsequent Evaluations

The Glaucoma Suspect

A glaucoma suspect is someone who, for one or more reasons, is at higher than usual risk of developing glaucomatous optic nerve damage and visual deficiency and therefore warrants careful follow-up. The most common conditions are the following:

- Elevated IOP
- Large or asymmetric optic cups
- Presence of a disc margin splinter hemorrhage
- Unexplained visual field defect consistent with glaucoma
- Strong family history of glaucoma

When a patient has one or more of these findings but does not convincingly fulfill the requirements of glaucoma diagnosis as outlined earlier during the *initial* evaluations, he or she requires periodic follow-up to monitor for conversion from being a glaucoma suspect to having manifest glaucoma. The interval of follow-up and repeat testing is based on the risk of future visual loss if conversion to glaucoma indeed occurs. Some high-risk glaucoma suspects may benefit from presumptive IOP-lowering treatment.

Chapter 6 deals with the management of glaucoma suspects with elevated IOP. Chapter 7 discusses the evaluation and management of normotensive patients with nerve and/or field changes suggestive of glaucoma. Chapter 8 reviews the management of normotensive patients with abnormal angle findings. Those with a strong family history of glaucoma are discussed in Chapter 12.

From Glaucoma Suspect to Manifest Glaucoma

Glaucoma suspects should be monitored regularly to determine if they develop manifest glaucoma. If a suspect with a visual field defect corresponding to a RNFL defect is noted to have previously undetected, episodic IOP elevation, he/she is diagnosed with glaucoma. Other findings consistent with conversion to glaucoma include:

- A confirmed new defect in a previously normal visual field consistent with glaucomatous damage (HAP2 criteria part I, page 53),
- A confirmed deepening or expansion of a previously ambiguous visual field defect (HAP2 criteria part III, page 106),
- Progressive thinning of the circumpapillary RNFL consistent with a glaucomatous process (see discussion in Chapter 5, pages 102-103 for patients who can do fields, and page 121-124 for those who cannot),
- Progressive optic disc cupping, notching or rim thinning documented by serial stereoscopic disc photographs.

In addition, for treatment purposes we diagnose as having manifest glaucoma a normotensive glaucoma suspect who has a negative neuro-ophthalmic workup and advanced visual field loss such that any increment of worsening, if it occurs, may be symptomatically important.

Some consider glaucoma with low baseline IOP ("normal tension glaucoma") to be an entity distinct from high-pressure forms of glaucoma, while others consider it within the spectrum of other open angle glaucomas. Clinically, we find it helpful to conceptualize glaucoma without elevated baseline IOP as a separate entity from high-pressure glaucoma as the natural history, evaluation strategy and clinical approach differ between the two, even though we believe that the two conditions represent the same disease. The following findings support glaucoma as the explanation of disc and field findings for which another explanation is not apparent:

- A high-normal pressure, perhaps 18 to 20 mmHg (rather than 12 to 15 mmHg) on the average;
- Typical glaucomatous configuration to the excavation of the nerve;
- Bilaterality of nerve fiber bundle defects in the visual field that do not respect the vertical meridian;
- A peripapillary crescent or halo on the disc margin;
- A splinter hemorrhage at the disc margin;
- Migraine, other forms of vasospasm, or low blood pressure;
- Family history of glaucoma;
- Significant myopia.

When optic nerve damage is present, the lower the accompanying IOP, the greater the suspicion for nonglaucomatous processes. Conversely, there is no way to completely rule out a nonglaucomatous process even in a patient who presents with elevated IOP and functional/structural changes classic for glaucoma. We recommend neuro-ophthalmologic testing when a patient presents with glaucomatous-appearing optic nerve damage with low baseline IOP and any of the following [1] –

- Age < 50 years
- Best-corrected vision < 20/40 (unless explained by other clear findings on exam)
- Optic disc pallor greater than cupping
- Visual field with borderline vertical midline defect
- Headaches and/or localizing neurologic symptoms

A history of a major hemodynamic crisis favors the diagnosis of nonprogressive damage but does not rule out glaucoma. The approach to investigate and rule out nonglaucomatous optic nerve damage is discussed in Chapter 7, while the approach to evaluate possible intermittent IOP elevation that is not apparent during the initial evaluation is outlined in Chapter 2.

Classification of Degree of Visual Field Damage and Disease Stage

For discussion purposes, we refer to visual field defects as early, moderate, and severe. Of course, damage is a continuum, classes are artificial, and it is possible to find fields that do not seem to be properly classified by a given set of criteria. Since we will make management recommendations based on the degree of field loss, however, it seems appropriate to define terms. In practice, we usually look at a field and decide how it looks without a detailed, explicit determination of whether it "fits" into one or another category. Our general divisions are based on two criteria: overall extent of damage and proximity to fixation of damage. A small, dense, central defect weighs more heavily than does a somewhat large but just as dense peripheral defect. Examples of fields we would classify into each group follow, in addition to some definitions. In all cases it is assumed that the only cause of field loss is glaucoma and that the field test being interpreted is a Humphrey Central 24-2 threshold test with a size III stimulus.

Degree of Visual Field Damage

Part II of the HAP2 criteria for visual field interpretation provides a classification scheme for the degree of visual field damage (see box in page 64). In general, we use the HAP2 criteria classification for risk stratification during clinical care, and refer to International Classification of Diseases, 10th edition (ICD-10) disease stage categories for financial claims purposes (see section below). It is important to note that the degree of visual field damage may not always agree with disease stage, such that a patient with "severe stage glaucoma" with visual defects in both the superior and inferior hemifields may in fact have an early visual field defect as defined by HAP2 criteria part II. **The clinical decisions outlined in this book are based on the severity of visual field defects outlined by HAP2 criteria part II.**

Disease Stage Coding in the United States

Since the first edition of this book, disease staging has gained popularity and has been incorporated into the ICD-10. In general, these stages define the extent of glaucomatous disease for a particular patient, while HAP2 criteria define the degree of visual field defect for a particular eye. The ICD-10 stages are –

1. Mild or early-stage glaucoma – pre-perimetric glaucoma (with a normal visual field).
2. Moderate-stage glaucoma – optic nerve abnormalities consistent with glaucoma and glaucomatous visual field abnormalities in one hemifield, and not within 5° of fixation.
3. Severe-stage glaucoma – optic nerve abnormalities consistent with glaucoma and glaucomatous visual field abnormalities in both hemifields and/or loss within 5° of fixation in at least one hemifield.
4. Indeterminate – optic nerve abnormalities consistent with glaucoma are present without available visual field data.

HAP2 Criteria, Part II
Classification of Glaucomatous Visual Field Defects in a 24-2 Examination

Early defect (Figure 3-1)
Damage should be neither extensive nor near fixation. <u>All three of the following conditions should be met</u>:

- The mean deviation (MD) index is > -6 dB.
- No point in the central 5° has a sensitivity < 15 dB.
- On the pattern deviation (PD) plot, fewer than 25% (1-12) of the points are depressed below the 5% level and fewer than 10% (1-4) points are depressed below the 1% level.

Severe defect (Figure 3-2 to 3-5)
<u>Any of the following</u> findings indicates severe field loss:

- The MD is < -12 dB.
- Any point in the central 5° has a sensitivity of 0 dB.
- There are points within the central 5° with sensitivity < 15 dB in both hemifields.
- On the PD plot, more than 50% (27+) of the points are depressed below the 5% level or more than 25% (14+) points are depressed below the 1% level.

Moderate defect (Figure 3-6)
Any field defect that is neither early nor severe. In other words, <u>at least one of the following</u> findings should be present:

- The MD is ≤ -6 dB but ≥ -12 dB.
- In only one hemifield, there are points in the central 5° with sensitivity < 15 dB; none of the central points has a sensitivity of 0 dB.
- On the PD plot, 25% or more but 50% or fewer (13-26) of the points are depressed below 5% level and 10% or more but 25% or fewer (5-13) of the points are depressed below the 1% level.

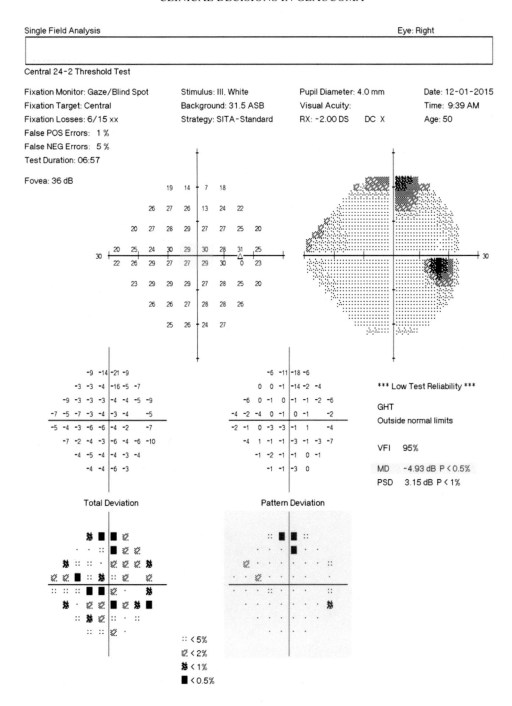

Single Field Analysis   Eye: Right

Central 24-2 Threshold Test

Fixation Monitor: Gaze/Blind Spot	Stimulus: III, White	Pupil Diameter: 4.0 mm	Date: 12-01-2015
Fixation Target: Central	Background: 31.5 ASB	Visual Acuity:	Time: 9:39 AM
Fixation Losses: 6/15 xx	Strategy: SITA-Standard	RX: -2.00 DS DC X	Age: 50
False POS Errors: 1 %			
False NEG Errors: 5 %			
Test Duration: 06:57			

Fovea: 36 dB

*** Low Test Reliability ***

GHT
Outside normal limits

VFI   95%

MD   -4.93 dB P < 0.5%
PSD 3.15 dB P < 1%

Total Deviation   Pattern Deviation

:: < 5%
✉ < 2%
✸ < 1%
■ < 0.5%

FIG 3-1. Early visual field defect by HAP2 criteria part II. The mean deviation (MD) index is less depressed than -6 dB. No point in the central 5° has a sensitivity of less than 15 dB. On the pattern deviation plot, fewer than 25% (13) of the points are depressed below 5% level and fewer than 10% (5) points are depressed below the 1% level (*yellow highlights*).

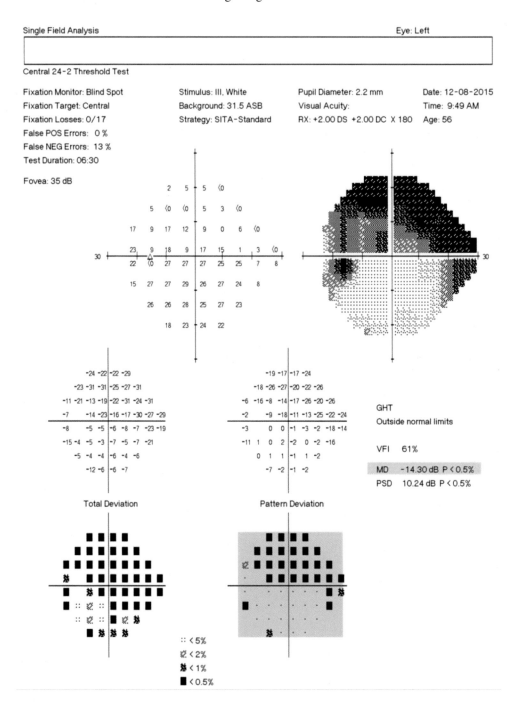

Single Field Analysis   Eye: Left

Central 24-2 Threshold Test

Fixation Monitor: Blind Spot   Stimulus: III, White   Pupil Diameter: 2.2 mm   Date: 12-08-2015
Fixation Target: Central   Background: 31.5 ASB   Visual Acuity: Time: 9:49 AM
Fixation Losses: 0/17   Strategy: SITA-Standard   RX: +2.00 DS +2.00 DC X 180   Age: 56
False POS Errors: 0 %
False NEG Errors: 13 %
Test Duration: 06:30

Fovea: 35 dB

GHT
Outside normal limits

VFI   61%

MD   -14.30 dB P < 0.5%
PSD   10.24 dB P < 0.5%

Total Deviation   Pattern Deviation

:: < 5%
⧖ < 2%
▨ < 1%
■ < 0.5%

FIG 3-2. Severe visual field defect by the HAP2 criteria part II. The mean deviation is worse than -12 dB, and more than 50% (25) of the points on the pattern deviation plot are depressed below the 5% level (*red highlights*)

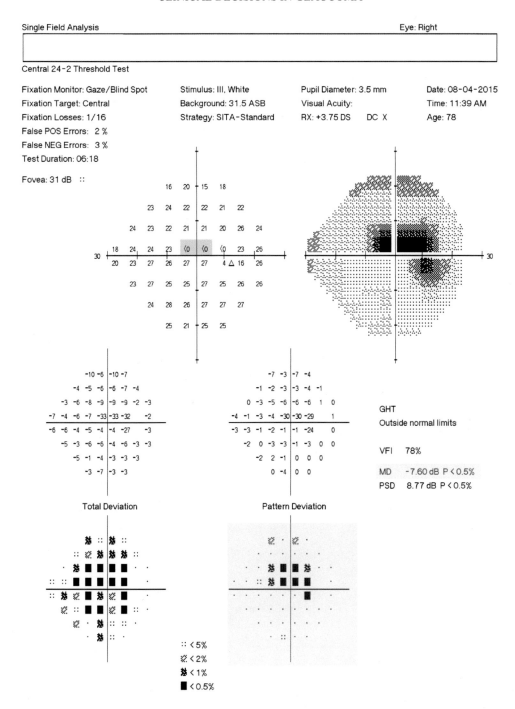

FIG 3-3. Severe visual field defect by the HAP2 criteria part II. At least one point in the central 5° has a sensitivity of 0 dB (*red highlight*). Note that the mean deviation and pattern deviation do not meet the criteria for severe defect (*yellow highlights*).

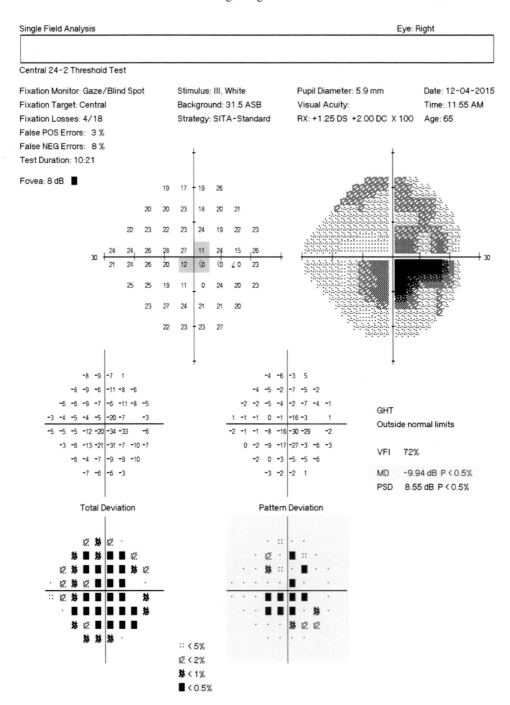

FIG 3-4. Severe visual field defect by HAP2 criteria part II. There are points within the central 5° with sensitivity < 15 dB in both hemifields (*red highlight*). Note that the mean deviation and pattern deviation do not meet the criteria for severe defect (*yellow highlights*).

Central 24-2 Threshold Test

Fixation Monitor: Gaze/Blind Spot	Stimulus: III, White	Pupil Diameter: 5.0 mm	Date: 07-21-2015
Fixation Target: Central	Background: 31.5 ASB	Visual Acuity:	Time: 8:14 AM
Fixation Losses: 1/16	Strategy: SITA-Standard	RX: +1.75 DS DC X	Age: 61

False POS Errors: 1 %
False NEG Errors: 6 %
Test Duration: 06:49

Fovea: 35 dB

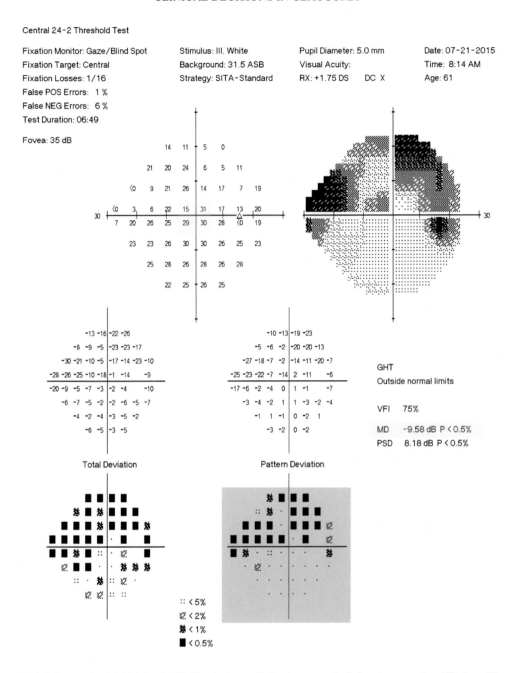

GHT
Outside normal limits

VFI   75%

MD   -9.58 dB P < 0.5%
PSD   8.18 dB P < 0.5%

Total Deviation

Pattern Deviation

:: < 5%
▨ < 2%
▩ < 1%
■ < 0.5%

FIG 3-5. Severe visual field defect by HAP2 criteria part II. On the pattern deviation plot, more than 50% (here 28) of the points are depressed below the 5% level and more than 25% (here 23) points are depressed below the 1% level. Note that the mean deviation was not worse than -12 dB (*yellow highlight*), nor are there any central points with sensitivity of < 15 dB (*yellow highlights*).

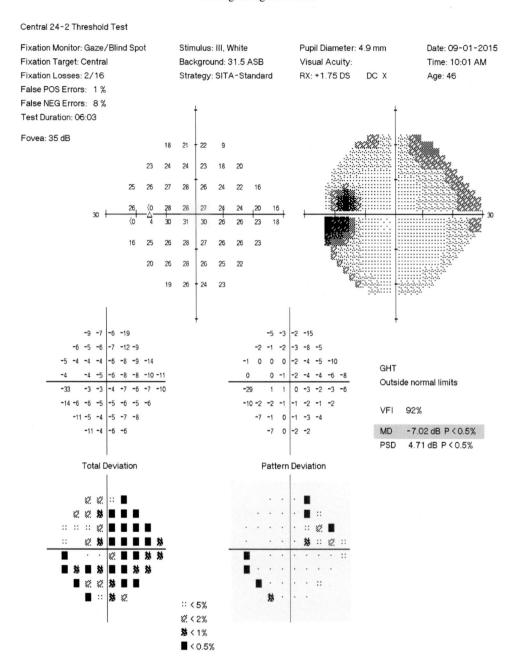

Central 24-2 Threshold Test

Fixation Monitor: Gaze/Blind Spot
Fixation Target: Central
Fixation Losses: 2/16
False POS Errors: 1 %
False NEG Errors: 8 %
Test Duration: 06:03

Fovea: 35 dB

Stimulus: III, White
Background: 31.5 ASB
Strategy: SITA-Standard

Pupil Diameter: 4.9 mm
Visual Acuity:
RX: +1.75 DS   DC X

Date: 09-01-2015
Time: 10:01 AM
Age: 46

GHT
Outside normal limits

VFI   92%

MD   -7.02 dB P < 0.5%
PSD   4.71 dB P < 0.5%

Total Deviation

Pattern Deviation

:: < 5%
⚠ < 2%
✸ < 1%
■ < 0.5%

FIG 3-6. Moderate visual field defect by the HAP2 criteria part II. The field does not meet criteria for early defect because mean deviation (*red highlight*) is more depressed than -6 dB. None of the central points has a sensitivity of < 15 dB, and there are fewer than 50% of the points (here 16) on the pattern deviation depressed below the 5% level (*yellow highlights*).

Reference

1. Greenfield DS, Siatkowski RM, Glaser JS, Schatz NJ, Parrish RK 2nd. The cupped disc. Who needs neuroimaging? Ophthalmology. 1998 Oct;105(10):1866-74.

4 INITIAL TREATMENT OF GLAUCOMA

Glaucoma is a chronic condition. Patients who have glaucoma do not get better; their visual function stays the same or worsens. Treatment does not make them feel better. The physician sees no dramatic cures and receives few immediate emotional rewards. The best treatment does not always work, and some people lose vision despite the clinician's best efforts. The picture is not uniformly gray, however. Most people with glaucoma have adequate vision for their needs throughout their lives. In addition, the management of glaucoma is conceptually straightforward. Attention to detail, careful follow-up, and appropriate treatments favorably affect the course of the disease.

There are five basic steps to follow in managing a patient with glaucoma:

1. Establish a good baseline.
2. Set a reasonable target for intraocular pressure (IOP).
3. Lower the pressure.
4. Follow up with the patient to see if the target pressure is maintained and if the glaucomatous damage progresses.
5. Modify the target pressure and treatment as indicated by the patient's course.

The first three steps should proceed promptly after diagnosis and together constitute the initial treatment of glaucoma, discussed in this chapter. The fourth and fifth steps are the chronic, ongoing steps and are discussed in Chapter 5.

The early care of patients with glaucoma involves frequent examinations. These multiple visits allow time for educating the patient about the irreversible nature of glaucomatous visual loss and the value of pressure reduction to avoid progressive damage. Between initial examinations, the patient may formulate new questions that require answers and may develop misconceptions that need clarification. The chronic nature of glaucoma care deserves emphasis from the start. Patient education may be the most important aspect of the chronic care of glaucoma because effective management depends not on the prescription of therapy, but on the use of therapy consistently and for a long time. Frequent early visits convey a sense of importance about the treatment regimen.

Establishing a Baseline

To determine whether a patient's condition is stable or is worsening over time, a precise knowledge of the patient's status at the beginning of treatment is needed. Most of the baseline data will have been gathered in the initial diagnostic evaluation, but further measurements may be needed. If possible, try to complete the baseline within the first 2 months. A good baseline includes information on the range over which IOP varies without treatment, the appearance of the angle, the status of the nerve and circumpapillary retinal nerve fiber layer, and the status of the visual field. Establishing such a baseline requires an initial investment of time, energy, and expense, but the investment is rewarded by making subsequent management decisions easier.

Intraocular Pressure

Intraocular pressure varies from day to day and over the course of the day, and the range within which the pressure varies is used to determine a target pressure. If possible, obtain at least three measurements before beginning treatment. The IOP measurements should be obtained at different times of day and on three different days if possible. In patients diagnosed with glaucoma without elevated baseline IOP, frequent and multiple baseline IOP measurements may uncover episodically high IOP. We do not check pressures outside ordinary office hours. If the patient can obtain records of previous pressures, he or she should do so.

Angle Appearance

The appearance and depth of the angle should be recorded. If the angle is narrow or closed, prior efforts to broaden or open the angle (such as iridotomy or iridoplasty) and their outcomes should be noted. Some procedures, such as selective laser trabeculoplasty, leave no visible signs, and may be unwittingly duplicated if prior interventions were not meticulously documented.

Optic Disc Imaging

Baseline imaging of the disc is discussed in Chapter 2.

Visual Fields

The baseline visual field examination is discussed in Chapters 2 and 3. Even a patient who has fully manifest glaucoma at the time of presentation should have at least two baseline field examinations to determine the variability of repeat threshold measurements. More than two sets of fields are sometimes needed to establish a baseline free of learning effects and artifacts; rarely, establishing the visual field baseline may extend over several months. If an individual continues to improve after the second or third examination, fields should be obtained on most visits until the field levels. There is no way to make the baseline field examination easy. However, to recognize subsequent change it is necessary to invest the time, energy, and money initially.

Setting an Initial Target Pressure

We used the term "pressure goal" in the first edition of this book to describe a management objective at which the benefits and risks of therapy favor the patient's overall long-term well-being. Hence, the formulation of a pressure goal takes into account the initial IOP, disease severity, rate of progression, patient's life expectancy, and the inconveniences and side effects of treatment. For example, if a patient is diagnosed with mild glaucoma and has a short projected life expectancy, the clinician may elect to observe the course of the condition and intervene only if it progresses more rapidly than predicted.

Since the publication of the first edition, the term "target pressure" has been popularized in glaucoma literature, and setting a target pressure is now considered a clinician performance quality measure. [1] The term "target pressure" has been defined as [2] –

1. The pressure at which the physician expects the rate of loss (of ganglion cells) to be no greater than the age-dependent rate, or

2. The highest IOP in a given eye at which the IOP does not contribute to the development of clinically apparent glaucomatous optic nerve damage.

In clinical practice, many doctors set "target pressures" for their patients using, at least in part, the criteria we previously described for choosing a pressure goal. For the purposes of this book, we have chosen to define "target pressure" as: *the upper limit of a range of IOP at which the clinician expects the rate of glaucomatous damage to be slowed sufficiently such that the patient is likely to preserve good vision for his or her lifetime.*

Since it denotes the upper limit of a range, **the target pressure will be higher than the desired average pressure**. In general, the more severe the disease, the narrower the allowed fluctuation. Given predicted stability around average IOP of x, a patient with early or moderate visual field defects may have target of $x+4$, while a patient with advanced disease may have target of $x+2$.

Setting the Target Pressure

Once the baseline is established, it is time to set an initial target pressure. Two useful concepts to help assess a given patient's risk of damage from elevated pressure are the estimated *threshold for damage* and the presence of *non-pressure risk factors*. In addition, the *extent of damage* already present determines, in part, the risk that additional damage will cause the patient noticeable visual disability and thus helps determine the importance of avoiding an increment of progression.

Threshold for damage. Assume that each patient has some IOP level below which there will be no glaucomatous damage. This pressure is the threshold for damage for that patient. The higher his or her IOP is above the threshold, the more rapidly glaucomatous damage will progress. Once the pressure falls below threshold, additional lowering of pressure provides no benefit and entails unnecessary risks. We cannot determine *a priori* a person's threshold for damage, but the findings at the time of presentation provide clues. We assume that an asymptomatic patient with elevated IOP has had high pressure for some time, and time has shown the susceptibility of his or her disc. Thus the extent of optic nerve and visual field damage that has already occurred yields some clue to the patient's susceptibility to damage. The greater the glaucomatous damage at the time of diagnosis, the more above threshold the pressure presumably is.

Non-pressure risk factors. This concept was introduced in Chapter 1. Some factors other than IOP determine why an individual develops glaucomatous damage at a particular pressure. The greater the degree of damage already present at diagnosis in a person with a given IOP, the more of these other risk factors that person is presumed to possess. And the greater the unknown risk factors, the more IOP should be lowered because it is the only treatable risk factor. Conversely, a person who, despite a distinctly elevated IOP, has minimal damage probably has few additional risk factors and may not need a profoundly low IOP to prevent further damage.

Extent of damage. The extent of damage is thus the major clue to the threshold for damage and to the presence of non-pressure risk factors. In addition, when setting a target pressure, the extent of damage determines the likely effect on the patient's useful visual function if he or she has progressive damage. In an eye with extensive nerve damage and field loss, each increment of structural damage causes more functionally critical loss than the same increment of damage causes in a less damaged eye. Thus the greater the damage, the greater should be the attempt to lower the IOP.

Specific Numbers

With these considerations in mind, set a target pressure for each patient. In the previous edition, we provided an intuitive, qualitative framework for setting a pressure goal based on the extent of damage on presentation and the presumed threshold for damage. In the subsequent two decades, data from several large, well-designed, multi-center clinical studies have supplemented this framework and provided guidance for setting initial target pressures. In particular, these studies provided the *mean* pressures at which the glaucomatous process was halted or too slow to detect in the study population. From this data, we can infer a reasonable *upper limit* of an IOP range within which the benefits and risks of therapy favor the patient's overall long term wellbeing. The guidelines for setting initial target pressures in manifest glaucoma are summarized below (Chart 4-1). The guidelines for setting an initial target pressure for a glaucoma suspect due to ocular hypertension, if therapy is appropriate, are discussed in Chapter 6.

Many target pressures suggested here will be higher than "normal," or conversely, will be considerably less than the upper limit of normal pressure. The fact that the target pressure does not respect the normal physiologic range in no way negates the importance of IOP lowering. In a given person, this suggested *initial* target pressure may represent too much or too little IOP lowering. Only over time will the answer be known. As the patient's course becomes apparent with subsequent follow-up, the target pressure may be modified (Chapter 5).

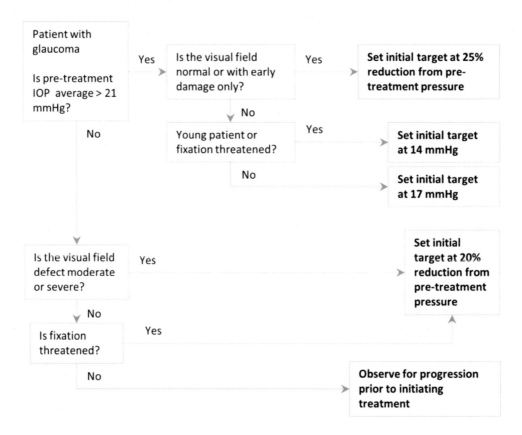

CHART 4-1. Setting an initial target pressure in manifest glaucoma. The target pressure is the **upper limit of a range of IOP** at which the clinician expects the rate of glaucomatous damage to be sufficiently slowed such that the patient is likely to preserve good vision for his or her lifetime, and thus is likely higher than the average IOP at which glaucoma progression stops. The severity of the visual field defect is based on HAP2 criteria part II (page 64).

Glaucoma with elevated average pre-treatment IOP. This group of patients has IOP > 21 mmHg most of the time and has either manifest glaucoma on initial evaluation as outlined in Chapter 3, or has converted from glaucoma suspect to glaucoma on follow-up by demonstrating progressive glaucomatous damage. The specific *initial target pressure* numbers are based on the extent of damage at diagnosis. The Comparison of Initial Glaucoma Treatment Study[3,4] and the Advanced Glaucoma Intervention Study yielded valuable data relating visual field progression and pressure achieved with therapy. Based on these data, we recommend the following: *

---

* The Comparison of Initial Glaucoma Treatment Study found that for patients with average visual field mean deviation of -4.8 dB, a 37% reduction in IOP with medication or laser resulted in no net visual field progression in 5 years. [3, 4] A *post hoc* analysis of the Advanced Glaucoma Intervention Study showed that in patients with average mean deviation of -10.5 dB, those with IOP lowered (by surgery and/or laser) to < 18 mmHg on all visits (average 12.3 mmHg) had no net progression over 8 years, while those with 75-99% of visits < 18 mmHg (average IOP of 14.7 mmHg) lost an average of 2.3 dB over 8 years. [5,6]

Pre-perimetric disease or early glaucomatous visual field loss – set target at 25% reduction from pre-treatment pressure.

Moderate to severe glaucomatous visual field loss – if fixation is threatened or lost, or if the patient has a long life expectancy, set target at 14 mmHg. If the fixation is spared or if the patient has a modest life expectancy, set target at 17 mmHg.

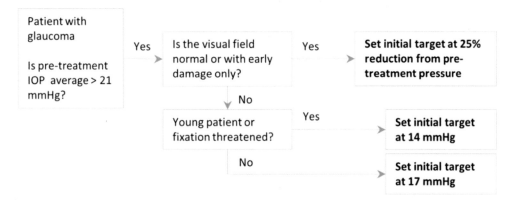

Glaucoma without elevated average pre-treatment IOP. Most of these patients, after initial evaluation, will carry a diagnosis of glaucoma suspect (Chapter 7), until progressive structural/functional changes declare the presence of glaucoma (Chapter 3). The Collaborative Normal Tension Glaucoma Study provided valuable insight into the natural history and management outcomes of these patients.* Based on this study, we recommend the following:

Early glaucomatous visual field loss AND fixation not threatened – observe for progressive changes and conversion from suspect to manifest glaucoma prior to initiating treatment (Chapter 3).

Moderate to severe glaucomatous visual field loss OR fixation threatened – set target at 20% reduction from pre-treatment pressure.

---

* In a *post hoc* analysis of patients who did not receive ocular hypotensive therapy (the observation arm of the study and patients observed but not enrolled in the study), 55% showed no progression after a mean follow-up of 5.6 years. In this group, the average initial mean deviation was -5.9 dB and 31% of the patients had threatened fixation. In the treatment arm, 80% of the patients showed no progression. The average initial mean deviation was -8.38 dB and 63% had threatened fixation. Treatment to achieve 30% reduction of mean IOP (with medication, laser or surgery) decreased the 5-year risk of visual field progression from 60% to 20%. [7]

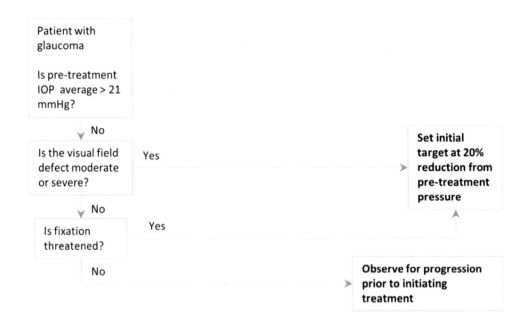

Treatment Approaches to Lower IOP

Therapeutic Options

Once a target pressure has been determined for a patient, institute therapy to try to achieve the target. By this time, in appropriate patients, any pupillary block component should have been alleviated by the performance of an iridotomy. It is currently assumed – although possibly not true – that the beneficial effect of lowering IOP is independent of how the lowering is achieved. That is, we treat glaucoma as if the nerve does not care if the pressure is 14 mmHg because of a drop, a pill, a laser treatment, or surgery. Each treatment has different side effects, and the appropriate order in which to institute therapies is a subject of ongoing dispute. The three major suggested courses are the following:

- Start with topical monotherapy. If this is ineffective, either perform laser trabeculoplasty or add additional topical agents. If the IOP remains too high, add more topical agents or do laser surgery, whichever has not been tried. If the pressure is still too high, systemic carbonic anhydrase inhibitor therapy and/or incisional surgery may be indicated.
- Perform laser trabeculoplasty first. If the pressure is not low enough, add topical monotherapy. If the pressure remains too high, add more topical and/or systemic agents. If this is not sufficient, incisional surgery may be indicated, depending on disease severity. Laser is not a first choice option in patients with synechial angle closure or other contraindications to laser trabeculoplasty.
- Perform incisional surgery first. The next steps if the surgery is ineffective are generally not specified.

For each of these courses, reasonable supporting and opposing arguments exist. Some of the major points regarding each approach are summarized as follows.

Medicine first, laser second, incisional surgery third –

Supporting arguments. This is the most commonly followed, traditional course. Easily tolerated topical medications lower pressure in most patients. Medications can be stopped or altered easily, and unlike either laser or incisional surgery, topical medications rarely cause acute ocular complications. The most severe systemic reactions (asthma, congestive heart failure) occur rarely; taking a good medical history usually alerts the physician to a patient's risk for such problems. If topical monotherapy fails to achieve the pressure goal after a short time, laser trabeculoplasty or addition of other topical agents often lowers pressure enough. If both medication and laser fail, incisional surgery can always be performed.

Drawbacks. Ocular medications can be expensive and bothersome to use. Many people are unable or unwilling to use them regularly. When the patient misses a dose or takes a dose late, the pressure may rise and nerve damage may occur. All topical therapies have side effects. When people must use drops daily, their quality of life suffers, and they are constantly aware of their disease. Topical medications may promote changes in the conjunctiva that limit the success of subsequent filtering surgery.

Laser first, medicine second, incisional surgery third –

Supporting arguments. Laser trabeculoplasty safely lowers the IOP in most people who have chronic open angle glaucoma. It may eliminate, reduce, or postpone the need for topical medications. After treatment, laser surgery causes no daily nuisance and requires no compliance except for routine follow-up visits. Laser exerts its effect 24 hours a day. Thus when successful, laser therapy obviates constant, day-in, day-out, attention. If laser surgery proves ineffective, then topical or systemic medications can still be used. Laser treatment has not been shown to limit the success of subsequent incisional surgery.

Drawbacks. Laser trabeculoplasty is often a temporary treatment that loses its effect over time. Most people treated initially with the laser require medications, and the laser provides only a fairly short reprieve. It may cause IOP elevations that may damage the eye. In the rare event that the IOP is actually raised instead of lowered, the patient may require surgery that he or she would otherwise have avoided.

Incisional surgery first –

Supporting arguments. After a successful procedure, the patient leads a fairly normal life and usually visits the eye doctor less frequently than do glaucoma patients treated in other ways. In some instances, successful surgery achieves pressures lower than can be obtained with medications and the pressure control is full time. Since the first edition of this book, the options for incisional glaucoma surgery have increased. It has been recognized that routine, clear-corneal phacoemulsification often lowers IOP for several years,[8] while numerous conjunctiva-sparing procedures (many of which are based on the principle of trabecular bypass) offer alternatives to traditional filtering surgery or glaucoma drainage device (GDD) implantation. If bleb-forming surgery precedes topical therapy, the success rate of trabeculectomy may be higher than reported for patients treated medically first, because eye drops cause irritation and conjunctival changes. If surgery fails, medications and lasers may then be tried. Incisional surgery costs more than other treatments initially, but over time surgery may be less expensive because of fewer doctor visits and reduced medication expenses.

Drawbacks. Surgery is not always successful, and successful surgery may fail after several years, a relatively short time in relation to the patient's life. Intraocular surgery carries a risk of infrequent but immediate, severe, potentially-blinding complications. The presence of a bleb places the patient at an ongoing increased risk of endophthalmitis. Glaucoma surgery speeds up cataract development. Previously-successful surgery may fail after cataract extraction. If surgery were to be done as the usual initial treatment for patients with primary open angle glaucoma, it would place many patients who would do very well with less risky management at risk for these complications.

Suggested Approach

For treatment-naïve patients with open angles and no contraindication to laser, we believe either medication or trabeculoplasty is a reasonable first step. Our general management course for glaucoma is as follows:

1. Initial treatment –
   - Topical therapy used once or twice a day (single medication or fixed-dose combinations) or laser trabeculoplasty
   - Choice (laser or topical therapy) not tried first
2. Modification of initial treatment –
   - Topical therapy with side effects that are tolerable
   - Non-bleb forming incisional surgery, if appropriate
   - Systemic carbonic anhydrase inhibitor therapy, if well tolerated
   - Bleb-forming incisional surgery (filter or GDD)

Most of our patients choose to start treatment with topical therapy. We quickly determine if a patient will easily achieve satisfactory pressure control with well-tolerated topical therapy. We prefer not to encourage forbearance with a regimen of multiple medications and move quickly to laser treatment or to do incisional surgery.

Laser Trabeculoplasty

The technique of laser trabeculoplasty is described in standard glaucoma textbooks. We treat 180° of a patient's angle in one sitting. If the patient's pressure remains above the target pressure 6 weeks after laser trabeculoplasty, then we treat the remaining 180°. If the patient's pressure remains above the target pressure 6 weeks after all the angle has been treated, then the decision must be made whether to proceed with additional pressure lowering or to observe for stability.

Principles of Topical Therapy

Several general principles contribute to the goal of maximizing the therapeutic effect of each topical medication while minimizing side effects. These principles are:

1. **Start with the least offensive drug first.** This is a subjective judgment. The considerations include ocular and systemic side effects, cost, and dosage frequency.
2. **Encourage lid closure after drop use.** Gentle lid closure for several minutes after drop use increases the contact time between the eye drops and the cornea by removing the lacrimal pumping action of the blink. More medication enters the eye and less medication enters the systemic circulation because there is less drainage onto the nasal mucosa via the nasolacrimal duct. Nasolacrimal duct obstruction for several minutes is an alternative if the patient has difficulty controlling his or her blinking.
3. **Use as few medications as possible.** Two separate medications are more difficult to use regularly than one single medication or a fixed-dose combination. Medicine that is used four times a day is less desirable than medicine that is required only once or twice a day.
4. **If more than one drop is used, allow time for each drop to be absorbed.** The cul-de-sac holds less than one drop. If a patient instills two different drops, one immediately after the other, one of two things happens. Either the second drop washes the first one out (and onto the cheek, where it is wasted, or into the lacrimal system, where it enters the systemic circulation), or the two drops mix and dilute one another. Because the amount of drug absorbed into the eye relates to its concentration, such a mix is less effective than the two drugs separated by enough time for the first to be absorbed. The ideal spacing for drops depends on a variety of variables, particularly the patient's rate of blinking. We assume that many patients reduce our time recommendations and thus suggest 10 minutes in the hope of achieving at least 5 minutes of separation.
5. **Give the patient written instructions.** It is not easy for calm, medically sophisticated people to remember medication instructions. Anxious patients often completely misunderstand or forget directions.

Outflow Pressure and Glaucoma Medication

Conventional outflow. In addition to following these guidelines, it is useful to have a general expectation of the effects of various drug treatments. Understanding the concept of outflow pressure is helpful. Glaucoma medications either decrease the amount of aqueous humor formed or decrease the resistance to the outflow of aqueous humor. Medications do not lower pressure by a fixed amount, nor do they lower pressure by a fixed percentage. For example, a particularly effective drug that reduces aqueous humor formation by 50% will not lower the pressure by 50%, but will lower it halfway from the starting pressure toward the episcleral venous pressure. Thus if episcleral venous pressure is 10 mmHg, a pressure of 20 mmHg will be lowered halfway toward 10 mmHg, resulting in a pressure of 15 mmHg (a 25% decrease). Similarly, a pressure of 30 mmHg will be lowered to 20 mmHg (halfway to 10 mmHg), a 33% lowering. A pressure of 40 mmHg will fall 38% to 25 mmHg, etc.

If the pressure is already lowered by one drug, both the percent and magnitude of pressure decrease from a second, equally effective drug (one that provides another 50% lowering of aqueous humor production) will be less than the first. The first drug may lower the pressure 10 mmHg from 30 mmHg to 20 mmHg, whereas the second achieves only an additional 5 mmHg decrease, from 20 mmHg to 15 mmHg. The following example illustrates the concept of outflow pressure.

Assumptions –
Negligible uveoscleral outflow
Episcleral venous pressure is 10 mmHg
Drug A decreases outflow pressure by 40%
Drug B decreases outflow pressure by 33%

Pre-treatment IOP	40 mmHg	30 mmHg	20 mmHg
Outflow pressure	30 mmHg	20 mmHg	10 mmHg
Effect of A	*12 mmHg*	*8 mmHg*	*4 mmHg*
IOP after A	28 mmHg	22 mmHg	16 mmHg
(New outflow pressure)	(18 mmHg)	(12 mmHg)	(6 mmHg)
Effect of B	*6 mmHg*	*4 mmHg*	*2 mmHg*
IOP after A + B	22 mmHg	18 mmHg	14 mmHg
% reduction after A + B	45%	40%	30%

With the same two drugs, the patient with the initial pressure of 40 mmHg will have a decrease of 18 mmHg and the patient with initial pressure of 20 mmHg will have a decrease of 6 mmHg. This example demonstrates two points about how much effect to expect from medication:

- The higher the initial pressure, the greater the decrease in pressure for a given medicine.
- The first drug used will probably provide the greatest numerical change in pressure.

Uveoscleral outflow. Also known as *pressure-independent outflow*, uveoscleral outflow occurs when aqueous passes from the anterior chamber into the suprachoroidal spaces via the ciliary muscle. It has been estimated to account for 5-15% of total aqueous outflow.[9]

Prostaglandin analogs increase uveoscleral outflow and may be synergistic with medications that either decrease aqueous production or increase conventional outflow.

Treating to Lower the Pressure: Specifics

We most commonly begin treatment with either a beta-blocker or a prostaglandin analog, usually after a discussion with the patient regarding each agent's potential side effects. In general, the following guidelines apply:

- Use the agent that has fewer relative contraindications.
- If only unilateral treatment is needed in a patient with lightly colored irides, avoid prostaglandin analogs.
- If the patient has multiple systemic diseases, or is on a systemic beta-blocker, a prostaglandin analog is preferred.

We no longer use a monocular trial of medications to gauge potential pressure-lowering effect, although we occasionally use one to gauge potential side effects. [10]

Prostaglandin analog as first medicine. In 2016, there are four prostaglandin analogs available in the United States as topical therapy for glaucoma: latanoprost, bimatoprost, travoprost and tafluprost. Unoprostone is no longer commercially available in the United States. When selecting a prostaglandin analog as first medicine, the physician should be mindful of its relative pressure-lowering effect, formulation, and cost.

Relative pressure-lowering effect. When dosed once nightly, latanoprost 0.005%, travoprost 0.004%, tafluprost 0.0015% and bimatoprost 0.03% or 0.01% have similar efficacy and are all superior to unoprostone 0.15%.

Formulation. Latanoprost and bimatoprost are both preserved with benzalkonium chloride, while travoprost is preserved by a trademarked preservative containing boric acid, propylene glycol, sorbitol and zinc chloride. Tafluprost is exclusively marketed as preservative-free. In patients who have demonstrated intolerance to benzalkonium chloride, travoprost or tafluprost may be tolerated.

Cost. Latanoprost and travoprost are available in generic formulations. They are likely to be less expensive than brand name medications.

Beta-blocker as first medicine. The following considerations apply to the decision of which beta-blocking agent to use first in a given patient: selectivity, relative pressure-lowering ability, and formulation (solution vs. suspension).

Selectivity. Timolol and levobunolol are nonselective (beta-1 and beta-2) blockers; betaxolol is a cardioselective (beta-1) blocker. The nonselective blockers, in addition to decreasing aqueous production, also increase airway resistance and decrease the cardiac output and the cardiac response to exercise. These drugs may precipitate asthma, respiratory failure, and congestive heart failure. Betaxolol has substantially less effect on the bronchial smooth muscle than nonselective drugs, and thus causes fewer respiratory complications than others. Betaxolol does have some effect on respiratory muscle, and it has been associated with respiratory complications.

Relative pressure-lowering effect. Timolol and levobunolol are slightly more effective in lowering IOP than is betaxolol.

Formulation. All the beta-blockers are available in solutions. In addition, timolol is available as a gel-forming solution, which, when applied once daily, lowers IOP equally to timolol solution dosed twice daily. Betaxolol is also available as a suspension. Particles in the suspension remain in the cul-de-sac and thus available to enter the eye longer than does the medication in solution, and the ocular effect of betaxolol 0.25% suspension is equivalent to betaxolol 0.5% solution. This ocular equivalence results in a lower systemic dose per unit of ocular dose. Suspensions must be shaken, however, to ensure that the concentration is accurate.

When treating an individual who has respiratory or cardiac disease, we consult with the patient's primary care provider before prescribing a beta-blocker unless the patient is already taking a beta-blocking agent. In this case, we assume that the internist would approve of using topical beta-blockers. However, in such individuals, the eye may already be partially treated with a beta-blocker, and topical therapy may achieve little. If the patient is not using a systemic beta-blocker and if a trial of selective beta-blocker treatment is considered safe, we order betaxolol suspension. We begin therapy in one eye at a time, and the patient is cautioned to notify us promptly of any changes in his or her medical status. Before treating the second eye, we ask specifically about symptoms because bilateral treatment doubles the systemic dose.

After choosing a beta-blocker, the clinician must decide how frequently the patient should use it. Twice daily usage is traditional and covers occasional missed doses, but once daily may be sufficient. If once daily treatment is chosen, we advise the patients to use it immediately on arising in the morning, because beta-blockers have little or no effect on aqueous formation during sleep.

Evaluation and Modification of Initial Treatment

Evaluation after Initial Treatment

If possible, obtain at least three baseline IOPs at different times of day prior to initiating treatment. After instituting treatment to the eye(s), the next step is to determine its effectiveness in lowering the IOP. The initial treatment and the extent of the patient's disease determine the timing of follow-up. Beta-blockers lower the IOP promptly, but the pressure may take some weeks to stabilize and usually does so at a higher pressure than that which immediately follows the initial dose. Thus the clinician can conclude quickly (in a day or two) that beta-blockers are inadequate, but it may take a month or two to be certain that an initially lowered IOP will remain adequately low to move on to chronic follow-up. Prostaglandin analogs lower IOP 3-4 hours after administration, although side effects sometimes do not become apparent until after 1-2 weeks of use. If the patient has very high pressure and significant damage, we may check the pressure the next day. It is usually possible to determine quickly if the first drug, or indeed full medical therapy, will be insufficient in such cases. However, if medical therapy is initially adequate, it is impossible to tell immediately if medical therapy will be sufficient over the longer term without examining the patient a month or so later. The effect of laser trabeculoplasty becomes apparent in about 6 weeks.

When the patient returns for assessment of initial therapeutic effect, the following determinations should be made:

Medication chosen as initial therapy –

- Determine if the patient is both taking and tolerating the medication. Ask whether the patient understood the directions and exactly how he or she is using the medication. Ask specifically if the patient has had side effects or any significant change in medical status. Record when the patient last took his or her medicine.
- Determine if the medication is lowering the pressure at all; if not, stop it. This is much easier if the pre-treatment average IOP is well-established with multiple visits. It is an unnecessary nuisance, risk, and expense to use a drug that has little or no effect.
- If the medication is lowering the pressure, decide if it is lowering it enough and modify treatment accordingly.

Laser chosen as initial therapy. Determine if the laser is lowering the pressure at all at 6 weeks. If not, treat the remaining 180° of angle and evaluate at 6 weeks.

Target pressure achieved. If the target pressure has been achieved, have the patient return for follow-up as described in Chapter 5.

Target pressure not achieved. If laser trabeculoplasty is effective but does not achieve a low enough pressure, initiate medical therapy. If the initial topical therapy is effective but does not achieve a low enough pressure, offer trabeculoplasty. If the patient declines laser treatment, substitute or add topical therapy.

Substitutions. If it seems reasonable to change rather than to add medication, we simply switch from a prostaglandin analog to a beta-blocker and vice versa.

Additions. If a beta-blocker alone is insufficient, either use the beta-blocker once daily and add a prostaglandin analog once nightly, or switch to a fixed-dose combination of two medications (e.g. dorzolamide/timolol). If a prostaglandin analog alone is not sufficient, add a beta-blocker used once daily (in the morning). If beta-blockers are contraindicated, add a topical carbonic anhydrase inhibitor.

After initial treatment with topical and/or laser therapies, decide if the pressure is close enough to the target to accept it. Given the imprecise nature of the target pressure, a pressure slightly (2 or 3 mmHg) above a patient's target may be acceptable in a patient with mild disease. In this case, move to the follow-up phase (Chapter 5). If the pressure is too high, especially if the disease is moderate or severe, other well-tolerated topical mediations may be added.

Modification of Initial Treatment

When full, well-tolerated, topical and laser therapies lower the pressure to some degree but do not decrease the pressure to target, there are two options: progress to additional treatment or observe the patient for stability. The choices for additional treatment are, in order of preference, additional marginally-tolerated topical therapy, non-bleb forming incisional surgery, systemic carbonic anhydrase inhibitors, and bleb-forming incisional surgery (filtration surgery and GDD implantation). Incisional surgeries that spare the conjunctiva and do not result in blebs may be offered to some patients who have failed well- tolerated topical therapy, especially if concurrent cataract surgery is planned.

Tolerated, even if not well-tolerated, topical therapy. For those patients who had bothersome but not intolerable side effects from one or more types of drops, another trial of topical therapy may be reasonable before considering systemic carbonic anhydrase inhibitors or incisional surgery. Fixed-dose combination medications (e.g. dorzolamide/timolol, brinzolamide/brimonidine) can increase tolerability by decreasing both the preservative load and the burden of administering multiple medications.

Systemic carbonic anhydrase inhibitors. Despite their sometimes severe and rarely life-threatening complications, systemic carbonic anhydrase inhibitors remain a useful group of drugs. We begin treatment with methazolamide 25 mg twice daily; if necessary, we increase the dosage to 50 mg twice or three times daily. If the pressure is still too high and the patient tolerates methazolamide, we change to acetazolamide 250 mg four times daily or to Diamox Sequels twice daily. Unless there is a compelling reason to avoid incisional surgery, we discontinue these medications in individuals with drowsiness, depression, renal stones, or other significant side effects. Like other sulfonamides, carbonic anhydrase inhibitors rarely cause blood dyscrasias of varying severity, including fatal aplastic anemia.* There has been some controversy about whether individuals treated with such medications should have regular complete blood counts performed. Recommendations regarding blood tests involve questions of the standard of care, the cost-benefit ratio of early detection of abnormalities, and the incidence and timing of carbonic anhydrase inhibitor-associated dyscrasias. It is currently not known how frequently – if ever – early recognition of a carbonic anhydrase inhibitor-related blood dyscrasia and prompt drug withdrawal improves the ultimate outcome of the condition. In the absence of better information, it seems reasonable to communicate any plans for systemic carbonic anhydrase inhibitor therapy with the patient's primary care provider, and to instruct the patient to report systemic symptoms.[11] Other side effects of systemic carbonic anhydrase inhibitors, such as metabolic acidosis,

---

* One study estimates the relative risk of aplastic anemia when taking acetazolamide to be 13.3, with an estimated incidence of approximately one in 18,000 patient-years.[10]

hypokalemia and renal calculi formation, should be kept firmly in mind when prescribing this group of medications.

Incisional surgery. Incisional glaucoma surgery is well described in standard surgical texts. For a patient with a visually significant cataract and chronic open angle glaucoma or some types of angle closure glaucoma, cataract extraction by phacoemulsification alone may lower the IOP to within the target range, although a glaucoma procedure (trabeculectomy, GDD implantation, or a conjunctiva-sparing trabecular bypass procedure) is sometimes performed concurrent with cataract extraction. The choice of procedure depends on the patient's extent of damage, the desired target pressure, and the surgeon's preference.

Evaluation for Additional Therapy: Algorithm

Chart 4-2 outlines our approach to the newly diagnosed glaucoma patient in whom initial treatment fails to achieve the pressure goal.

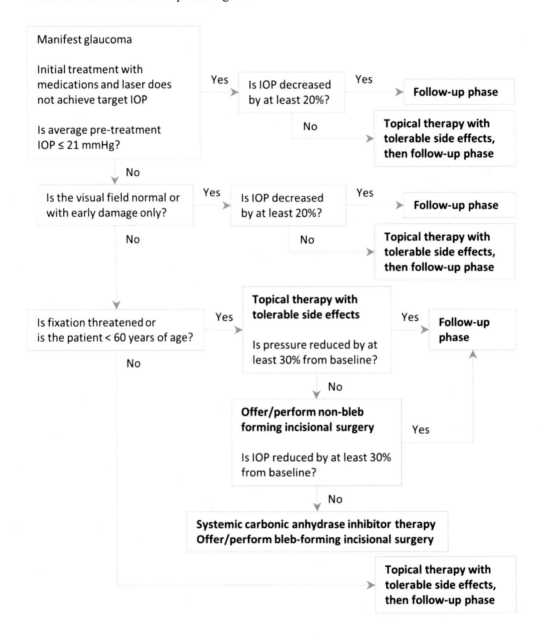

CHART 4-2. Approach when the target pressure is not achieved with initial therapy. Key – IOP (intraocular pressure).

Pre-treatment IOP ≤ 21 mmHg –

- If the IOP is at least 20% lower than the baseline, proceed to chronic follow-up.
- If the IOP is not lowered at least 20%, add topical therapy with tolerable side effects. Even if these steps do not achieve a 20% decrease in IOP, proceed with chronic follow-up to determine the pace of damage.

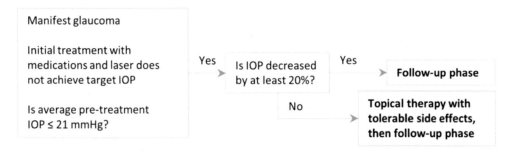

Pre-treatment IOP > 21 mmHg, pre-perimetric or early visual field damage –

- If the IOP is at least 20% lower than the baseline, proceed to chronic follow-up.
- If the IOP is not lowered at least 20%, add topical therapy with tolerable side effects. Even if these steps do not achieve a 20% decrease in IOP, proceed with chronic follow-up to determine the pace of damage.

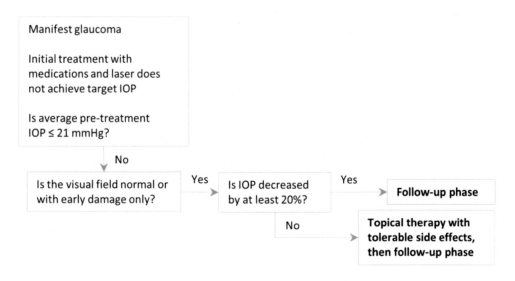

Pre-treatment IOP > 21 mmHg, moderate to severe visual field damage –

Young patient or fixation threatened – this group has the highest risk of losing useful vision given the disease severity and patient's life expectancy, and requires aggressive treatment.

- Add topical therapy with side effects that are tolerable.
- If the IOP is at least 30% lower than the baseline, regardless of whether the target is met, follow the patient's course.
- If the IOP is not lowered at least 30% on tolerated topical therapy, perform non-bleb forming surgery unless the patient declines.
- If surgery is successful and achieves at least a 30% decrease in IOP, proceed with chronic follow-up.
- If the IOP cannot be lowered at least 30%, start systemic carbonic anhydrase inhibitor therapy and consider bleb-forming incisional surgery.

Older patient and fixation not threatened.

- Add topical therapy with tolerable side effects.
- Follow the patient's course.

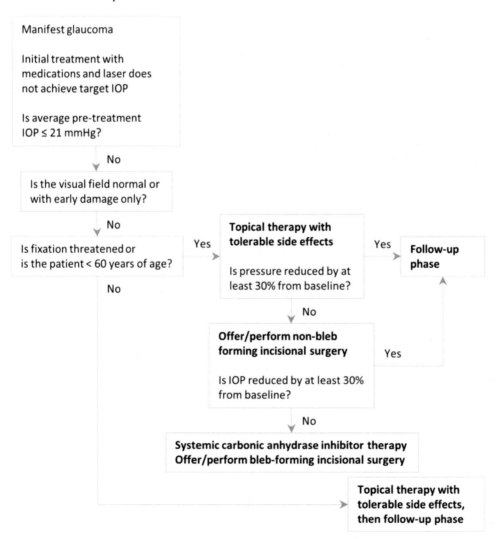

Treating to Lower the Pressure: Some Variations

Our recommended management of glaucoma presumes that clinicians can follow their patients over time and modify both target pressures and treatment as indicated by their courses. In some situations, however, it is difficult or impossible to assess further progression. The most common such clinical settings are as follows:

- The patient who cannot do reliable fields.
- The patient whose fundus cannot be seen well.
- The patient with far-advanced glaucoma on initial evaluation.

   The patient who cannot do reliable fields. If a patient cannot, despite education, perform reliable threshold visual fields, determine if the patient can perform any reliable fields. Suprathreshold testing is not as good as threshold testing, but if reliable it is better than nothing. In patients who cannot give good field information the disc examination and imaging assume greater importance. The greater the nerve damage, the more difficult it is to recognize a small change, and thus the more difficult it is to recognize progressive damage. If the optic nerve and circumpapillary retinal nerve fiber layer (RNFL) can be imaged precisely using optical coherence tomography (OCT), the following strategy can be used based on the OCT-RNFL analysis (Table 4-1):

- Normal thickness, normal contour – treat as a glaucoma suspect (Chapter 6, Glaucoma Suspect I: Ocular Hypertension)
- Normal thickness, abnormal contour – treat as early glaucomatous damage
- Borderline thickness, normal contour – treat as early glaucomatous damage
- Borderline thickness, abnormal contour, good vision – treat as moderate glaucomatous damage
- Borderline thickness, abnormal contour, poor vision – treat as severe glaucomatous damage
- Abnormal thickness, normal contour – treat as moderate glaucomatous damage
- Abnormal thickness, abnormal contour – treat as severe glaucomatous damage

TABLE 4-1. Assigning glaucoma severity based on retinal nerve fiber layer (RNFL) findings.

		Average overall RNFL thickness		
		Normal	*Borderline*	*Abnormal*
RNFL contour	*Normal*	Glaucoma suspect	Early glaucoma	Moderate glaucoma
	Abnormal	Early glaucoma	*Good vision* Moderate glaucoma / *Poor vision* Severe glaucoma	Severe glaucoma

The patient whose fundus cannot be seen well. In a patient whose fundus cannot be seen well because of miosis, cataract, or other media opacity, the visual field and pressure will be the key points to follow. In this case, set the target pressure based on the visual field severity classification outlined on page 64. The visual field constriction that usually accompanies small pupils and cataracts may lead to a low target pressure but in this situation it is reasonable. We have a low threshold to perform clear-corneal cataract surgery if the cataract precludes adequate fundus visualization.

The patient with far-advanced glaucoma on initial observation. Even if both the disc and field can be evaluated, the more severe an individual's glaucomatous damage already is at the time of diagnosis, the more difficult it is to recognize further change in either the disc or field. In addition, the more advanced a patient's glaucoma is, the greater the chance that damage will progress, and that a small additional amount of damage will cause symptomatically important worsening, such as loss of central fixation. If the disc and field are so badly damaged that further incremental damage will be difficult to recognize, we suggest the following arbitrary general guide:

1. Set a target IOP of 14 mmHg or 35% reduction, whichever is lower.
2. If the target IOP can be achieved, follow the patient's course carefully, as described in Chapter 5.
3. If this strict target cannot be achieved with medical or laser therapy –
    a. If the patient has two seeing eyes, do bleb-forming surgery on one of the eyes with a target of 12 mmHg.
    b. If the patient has only one seeing eye, do bleb-forming surgery if the pressure is either 20% above the target or is less than 30% below the baseline pressure.

The role of non-bleb forming glaucoma surgery is unclear in this group of patients, who often require drastic pressure-lowering beyond the effects typically achieved by these surgeries.

After completing the initial steps of management, glaucoma care moves into the chronic follow-up phase, described in Chapter 5.

References

1. American Academy of Ophthalmology Glaucoma Panel. Preferred Practice Pattern Guidelines. Primary Open angle Glaucoma. San Francisco, CA: American Academy of Ophthalmology; 2010. www.aao.org/ppp.

2. Jampel HD. Target pressure in glaucoma therapy. Journal of Glaucoma. 1997 Apr;6(2):133-8.

3. Collaborative Normal-Tension Glaucoma Study Group. The effectiveness of intraocular pressure reduction in the treatment of normal-tension glaucoma. Collaborative Normal-Tension Glaucoma Study Group. American Journal of Ophthalmology. 1998 Oct;126(4):498-505.

4. Collaborative Normal-Tension Glaucoma Study Group. Comparison of glaucomatous progression between untreated patients with normal-tension glaucoma and patients with therapeutically reduced intraocular pressures. Collaborative Normal-Tension Glaucoma Study Group. American Journal of Ophthalmology. 1998 Oct;126(4):487-97.

5. Palmberg P. How clinical trial results are changing our thinking about target pressures. Current Opinion in Ophthalmology. 2002 Apr;13(2):85-8.

6. Palmberg P. Evidence-based target pressures: how to choose and achieve them. International Ophthalmology Clinics. 2004 Spring;44(2):1-14.

7. Anderson DR, Drance SM, Schulzer M; Collaborative Normal-Tension Glaucoma Study Group. Natural history of normal-tension glaucoma. Ophthalmology. 2001 Feb;108(2):247-53.

8. Mansberger SL, Gordon MO, Jampel H, Bhorade A, Brandt JD, Wilson B, Kass MA; Ocular Hypertension Treatment Study Group. Reduction in intraocular pressure after cataract extraction: the Ocular Hypertension Treatment Study. Ophthalmology. 2012 Sep;119(9):1826-31.

9. Toris CB. Pharmacotherapies for glaucoma. Current Molecular Medicine. 2010 Dec;10(9):824-40.

10. Realini TD. A Prospective, randomized, investigator-masked evaluation of the monocular trial in ocular hypertension or open angle glaucoma. Ophthalmology. 2009 Jul;116(7):1237-42.

11. Keisu M, Wiholm BE, Ost A, Mortimer O. Acetazolamide-associated aplastic anaemia. Journal of Internal Medicine. 1990 Dec;228(6):627-32.

12. Mogk LG, Cyrlin MN. Blood dyscrasias and carbonic anhydrase inhibitors. Ophthalmology. 1988 Jun;95(6):768-71.

5 FOLLOW-UP OF GLAUCOMA PATIENTS

Establishing a baseline, setting an initial target pressure, and achieving the initial target pressure with treatment usually take a few months. The fourth and fifth steps in the management of glaucoma, following up on the patient's course and modifying treatment as indicated, continue for the patient's lifetime.

---

1. Establish a good baseline.
2. Set a reasonable initial target pressure.
3. Lower the pressure.
4. Continue to observe the patient to determine if the target pressure is met and if the glaucomatous damage progresses.
5. Modify the target pressure and treat as indicated by the patient's course.

Upon presentation, some patients will have had treatment initiated elsewhere without available information on pre-treatment intraocular pressure (IOP) or rate of deterioration. In these instances, it is helpful to ask the patient whether the previous clinician seemed to be dissatisfied with his or her pressure control and whether any changes were made recently. If not, and the patient has early glaucoma damage, it is appropriate to continue the same regimen and follow closely, provided that the regimen is well-tolerated. If, on the other hand, the patient recalls the clinician augmenting therapy, or if he or she has moderate or severe glaucomatous damage, treatment can be modified to reach the initial target pressure outlined in the previous chapter.

Patient Follow-Up

The underlying purpose of examining a patient with glaucoma on a regular basis is to improve the chance of preserving vision. The more prosaic reasons include monitoring the effects – both desired and undesired – of therapy, maintaining the patient's motivation to care for his or her disease, determining if the target pressure continues to be met, recognizing progressive damage, and modifying the target pressure and management, if needed, to achieve optimal visual preservation.

Three major questions arise in relation to follow-up:

- How frequently should the patient be examined?
- What should be tested at follow-up examinations?
- Is the patient's condition stable or worsening?

Frequency of Examinations

Specific follow-up examples appear in the following sections. In general, we see patients frequently in the first 2 or 3 years of their (recognized) disease, when we are uncertain of the pace of their condition and when they need to be reminded of the importance of continuous treatment. We examine patients with severe disease more frequently than those who have mild disease. We gradually lengthen the interval between examinations in patients whose conditions prove stable for 2 or 3 years.

These guidelines may translate into biweekly to monthly visits early in a patient's course, while the baseline is being established, a target is being set, and treatment is instituted to reach the target. Then the interval lengthens gradually to once or twice a year provided the patient's course remains stable. If the pressure becomes uncontrolled or if damage progresses, we evaluate the patient and modify management as necessary. We revert to more frequent visits and again slowly reduce the visit frequency.

Content of Follow-Up Examinations

History. Always take an interval history, particularly regarding possible side effects of medicine, changes in vision and/or general health, and medication adherence. Ask the patient to describe the schedule he or she is using for the treatment regimen; it may not correspond to the schedule prescribed.

Vision. Always check the visual acuity.

Intraocular pressure. Check the IOP in both eyes and record the time of measurement and time of last medication. Although patients do not always take every dose of their medication, most people do use their medicine before visiting the doctor. Thus an IOP measurement at or below the patient's target cannot ensure that the pressure is always low, but an IOP above the target generally indicates that the prescribed regimen does not reach the target pressure.

Gonioscopy. In the absence of unexpected IOP rise, we perform routine gonioscopy in phakic patients every 1-2 years after the initial evaluation because the angle configuration may change as the lens grows. If a miotic medication is used, examine the patient with a gonioprism soon after it has been added to the treatment regimen because miotics may narrow the angle in direct relation to their strength.

Fundus examination. Look for hemorrhages on the disc at every visit. Examine the disc with a lens that provides a magnified binocular view. As noted before, a Hruby lens or a contact lens may provide a better stereoscopic view than the 78D and 90D noncontact indirect fundus lenses. Use a slit beam to delineate the contour of the cup. In an undilated patient, it can be difficult to assess cupping, but disc hemorrhages can usually be seen on careful exam. In individuals with very small pupils or significant cataracts, a direct ophthalmoscope often provides a view of the nerve which is adequate to recognize blood. Dilate the patient's pupils at least once a year to compare the optic nerve to the baseline and to examine the fundus. When the pupil is dilated, examine the macula and the retinal periphery; glaucoma patients are susceptible to other eye conditions.

Retinal nerve fiber layer and optic disc imaging. Repeat the optical coherence tomography retinal nerve fiber layer (OCT-RNFL) analysis at least yearly in the first several years of follow-up. Progressive thinning of the overall RNFL or changes in RNFL contour from baseline in the absence of other pathology or study artifacts may indicate progression. In many patients, OCT-RNFL analysis of adequate signal strength can be acquired without dilation, but if dilation is planned we do the scan through the dilated pupil. A repeat set of stereoscopic disc photos is useful for side-by-side comparison to baseline photos if disc changes are suspected on examination. The comparison of new photographs to baseline photographs may be more sensitive in detecting glaucomatous change than comparing disc appearance on clinical examination with baseline photographs.

Visual fields. By the time most patients move into the follow-up phase of their care, they should have their field baseline established (Chapter 2). If a patient has significant variability or improves over the first four or five fields, obtaining the field baseline may extend into what is ordinarily the follow-up period. In such people, obtain a visual field test on most or all visits until a good, stable baseline is obtained.

Frequent fields early in the course of follow-up give a sense of the patient's variability and provide the opportunity to recognize unexpected rapid progression. If a series of several fields is stable over approximately 2 years, it is reasonable to extend the interval between field examinations, because the years of stability establish that if the patient is progressing at the achieved IOP, such progression is not rapid. If the pressure rises, if there are unexpected and confirmed changes on an OCT-RNFL analysis, or if a disc hemorrhage is noted on a visit when the patient does not have a field examination, we repeat the test promptly.

Follow-Up Planning Examples

The following hypothetical patient examples illustrate our recommendations for initial follow-up plans. How we decide whether the patient's condition is stable is discussed later; these examples outline our rationale about the frequency and nature of follow-up visits. Note that the frequency schedule and content of visits relate to the severity of the disease and length of patient follow-up. In general, to detect progression, structural examinations such as disc photos and OCT-RNFL are more useful in early glaucoma, while visual fields are more useful in moderate and severe glaucoma. Examine the nerve on every visit to detect any hemorrhages.

Case AB – easily controlled mild glaucoma. A 60-year-old asymptomatic woman is first seen with an IOP of 32 mmHg. Her cup/disc ratio is 0.5 and is concentrically enlarged slightly compared to excellent-quality optic disc photographs that the patient brought in, obtained elsewhere 4 years ago. Focal thinning is detected on OCT-RNFL analysis, and baseline static visual fields with excellent reliability are normal. Over three baseline exams completed within 2 months, untreated pressure measurements average 30 mmHg (range, 27 to 33 mmHg). The initial target is a 25% reduction from baseline (target 22.5 mmHg). Treatment with a beta-blocker in both eyes results in a pressure of 21 mmHg in both eyes after 1 month (3 months since her initial visit).

- When should this patient be reexamined?
- What should be tested on follow-up?

A patient who has only pre-perimetric glaucomatous damage despite a pressure in the high 20s to low 30s probably has a fairly high threshold for damage and probably has few non-pressure risk factors. Initially the focus is on whether the pressure remains below the target pressure and whether the patient tolerates the medication. It is reasonable to examine this person in a month or so to check the pressure. If it remains low, reexamine the patient again in 2 months (3 months into follow-up) to monitor the IOP. For this patient, glaucoma progression may manifest as progressive RNFL thinning, changes in RNFL contour, or a new scotoma in her previously normal visual field. If the patient's pressure remains at or below target, see the patient again in 3 months (6 months into follow-up) to test the IOP, perform another visual field and OCT-RNFL analysis, and dilate the patient's pupils to examine the disc and the rest of the fundus. If the visual field and OCT-RNFL analysis remain stable, check the pressure, perform gonioscopy, test the visual field and perform a dilated fundus exam and OCT-RNFL analysis in another 6 months (now 12 months into follow-up). Check the IOP and examine the disc in another 6 months, and perform gonioscopy, a visual field exam, an OCT-RNFL analysis, and a dilated fundus exam in 6 more months (24 months into follow-up). If the field and OCT-RNFL analysis remain stable 24 months into follow-up, and if the pressure remains within the target range, then continue to check the pressure every 6 months and perform field examinations and OCT-RNFL analyses yearly for 3 or 4 more years. Dilate the pupils and perform gonioscopy yearly. If the patient's condition is still stable after 5 years of follow-up, it is reasonable to examine the patient fully every 12 months. Table 5-1 summarizes the recommended routine baseline studies and follow-up schedules for individuals with mild disease.

Case CD – probably controlled moderate glaucoma. A 59-year-old man has untreated pressures that average 28 mmHg (range, 24 to 32 mmHg). His cup/disc ratio is 0.7 with a notch inferotemporally in both optic nerves and with corresponding superonasal moderate visual field defects sparing fixation that are consistent on two sets of baseline fields performed within 6 weeks of the initial visit. An OCT-RNFL analysis shows borderline mean RNFL thickness with marked inferior RNFL thinning. An initial target pressure is set at 17 mmHg. The patient has severe asthma, and his internist believes that beta-blocker use is contraindicated. Treatment with latanoprost results in pressures of 20 mmHg after a 2-week trial. Brimonidine produces intolerable symptoms after 1 day, and the patient is advised to use dorzolamide. One month later (3 months since presentation) the pressure is 16 mmHg in each eye.

- When should this patient be re-examined?
- What should be tested on follow-up?

This patient has significant disease, but he has responded nicely to medication. His threshold for damage is probably lower than that of patient AB, but he is unlikely to show measurable optic nerve or visual field changes after only a few months. The purpose of the initial follow-up examination is to ensure that the pressure remains low. Schedule a follow-up pressure check a month or so after achieving the initial target pressure. In 2 months (3 months into follow-up), check the pressure, repeat the visual field examination and ask carefully about side effects and assess adherence. Check the pressure in another 3 and 6 months, and at 12 months into follow-up, repeat tonometry, gonioscopy, visual field examination, dilated funduscopy and OCT-RNFL analysis. If the patient's condition remains stable, perform a visual field examination and monitor the pressure every 6 months and perform gonioscopy, dilate the pupils and repeat OCT-RNFL analysis yearly. If the field, OCT-RNFL and pressure remain satisfactory after five years, the visual field examination and OCT-RNFL could be done yearly and the pressure tested every 6 months. Table 5-1 summarizes the follow-up schedule for patients with moderate glaucoma.

Case EF – Marginally controlled severe glaucoma. A 64-year-old man with untreated pressures averaging 26 mmHg (range, 23 to 29 mmHg), has a cup/disc ratio of 0.85 with significant, fixation threatening visual field loss. Baseline fields are of good quality given the extent of damage, but there is a moderate amount of variation, particularly in the damaged areas. An OCT-RNFL analysis shows mean thicknesses of 50 and 60 microns. The target pressure is 14 mmHg. After he uses a beta-blocker for 2 weeks, the pressure measures 19 mmHg, and dorzolamide is added to both eyes. Two weeks later, the pressure is 15 mmHg. The patient is offered and promptly declines laser trabeculoplasty. Over the next month, with the subsequent addition of latanoprost to both eyes, his pressure is 13 mmHg. He is maintained on 3 agents – dorzolamide/timolol fixed-dose combination and latanoprost.

- When should this patient be reexamined?

- What should be tested on follow-up?

This patient has severe disease and a target pressure that has been barely attained. He probably has more non-pressure risk factors than the other two patients and thus has a lower threshold for damage. It may be difficult to recognize additional small increments of visual field loss in this patient with a fixation threatening defect on a standard 24-2 field due to the inherent variability of damaged fields. Because his RNFL is already very thin, progressive thinning may be difficult or impossible to recognize. Examine this patient in one month to check the pressure, ask about adherence, and perform a 10-2 visual field to better define his central field. If the pressure is still controlled, recheck the pressure and obtain a second baseline 10-2 visual field examination in another 2 months (3 months into follow-up). Check the IOP and repeat a 24-2 visual field in 3 more months (6 months into follow-up) and check the IOP again in 3 more months (9 months into follow-up). At 12 months into follow-up, repeat the pressure measurement, gonioscopy, dilated fundus exam, and 10-2 visual field examination. Thereafter, check the pressure and alternate 24-2 and 10-2 fields every 3 months for perhaps a total of 24 months. Repeat gonioscopy yearly if phakic. If the fields and pressures remain stable, the frequency of visits and fields may be decreased to every 6 months for another 2-3 years. Continue to examine the patient every 6 months and alternate between the 24-2 and 10-2 fields (Table 5-1).

TABLE 5-1. Follow-up schedules for patients with early, moderate and severe glaucomatous defects.

Baseline	• At least three IOP measurements at different times of day • At least two threshold visual field examinations (unless first examination is reliable and normal) • Gonioscopy • OCT-RNFL analysis • Disc photographs	Obtain within 2 months
Initial treatment	• Pressure checks and medication adjustment at 1- to 4-week intervals until treatment regimen is established	Complete within 3 months if possible
Follow-up	• See tables below	

Follow-up Phase of Early Glaucomatous Defect or Pre-Perimetric Glaucoma

										Years 3-5		After year 5
Months	1	3	6	9	12	15	18	21	24	q6 mos	q yr	q yr
IOP	x	x	x		x		x			x	x	x
Gonioscopy				x			x				x	x
Disc exam	x	x				x				x		
DFE		x		x			x				x	x
Visual field		x		x			x				x	x
OCT-RNFL		x		x							x	x
Disc photos	*Repeat if good quality OCT-RNFL cannot be obtained or if change is suspected*											

Follow-up Phase of Moderate Glaucomatous Defect

										Years 3-5		After year 5	
Months	1	3	6	9	12	15	18	21	24	q6 mos	q yr	q6 mos	q yr
IOP	x	x	x	x	x		x		x	x	x	x	x
Gonioscopy				x			x				x		x
Disc exam	x	x	x	x	x					x		x	
DFE				x			x				x		x
Visual field		x			x	x	x		x	x	x	x	x
OCT-RNFL					x		x				x		x
Disc photos	*Repeat if good quality OCT-RNFL cannot be obtained or if change is suspected*												

Follow-up Phase of Severe Glaucomatous Defect

										After year 3	
Months	1	3	6	9	12	15	18	21	24	q6 mos	q yr
IOP	x	x	x	x	x	x	x	x	x	x	x
Gonioscopy				x			x				x
Disc exam	x	x	x	x		x	x	x		x	
DFE					x				x		x
Visual field	x*	x*	x		x*	x	x*	x	x*	x*	x
OCT-RNFL	*Repeat only if a change might be recognizable*										
Disc photos	*Repeat only if a change might be recognizable*										

*10-2 visual field, repeat if it augments the 24-2 fields

Key – IOP (intraocular pressure), DFE (dilated fundus exam), OCT-RNFL (optical coherence tomography retinal nerve fiber layer analysis), q6 mos (every 6 months), q9 mos (every 9 months), q yr (yearly), q 1-2 yrs (every 1-2 years).

Recognition of Progressive Damage

Glaucoma rarely causes symptoms until it is very advanced; only in severe cases will the patient be able to tell the clinician that his or her vision is decreasing. Similarly, the visual acuity rarely alerts the clinician to deterioration because it does not decrease appreciably until glaucoma is profoundly advanced. Miotic use, especially in conjunction with cataract, may dim the vision or decrease the measured acuity.

To decide if a patient's condition is worsening or remaining stable over time, the clinician relies on the pressure, the appearance of the nerve, the OCT-RNFL analysis, and the visual field. The management of progressive damage is discussed beginning on page 112.

Pressure as a guide. Early in the course of glaucoma, the pressure offers mainly negative information. Regardless of how low the IOP is on a follow-up examination, a patient may undergo further damage either because of a low threshold for damage or because of variable compliance. But if the pressure measures consistently at a level known or reasonably presumed to be above the threshold, this information is useful. If the pressure rises into the range of the baseline IOP, assume that the eye is probably undergoing further damage. Any therapeutic decision based on pressure alone should be made only after pressure measurements on at least two occasions. Do not act on a single pressure reading that is out of line with the usual for the patient.

Optic nerve as a guide –

Cupping. The appearance of the optic nerve helps most in the chronic follow-up of patients with early to moderate glaucoma. Consider the role of the nerve photographs in the following hypothetical patient.

Case GH. In 2011 a 65-year-old patient is first seen by a clinician. The patient brings her records from the past 10 years of glaucoma care. There are 14 pages of photocopied and printed records; the pretreatment pressures in 2001 were 25 and 27 mmHg. With therapy the pressures have varied between 17 and 23 mmHg, with most readings approximately 19 mmHg. In 2001 the patient's nerves were described as "0.6." The clinician has copies of two sets of screening fields done on Frequency Doubling Technology type perimeters in two different offices, and the fields show variably plotted nerve fiber bundle defects. Two fields done on a Dicon perimeter, one field on an Octopus perimeter, and three fields on a Humphrey perimeter all show comparable abnormalities. The last three fields look as if they might be worsening, but the patient reports that over the past 4 years a cataract has been developing. Her vision, which was 20/20 in 2001, is now 20/40. However, her pupils dilate nicely and the clinician can obtain a good view of the nerves. She has a cup/disc ratio of 0.5 horizontally and 0.7 vertically with a notch inferotemporally in each eye. It is not known if her condition is currently stable. Then she shows the clinician photographs taken in 2001. If the photographs look like the nerves in 2011, the clinician can be confident that the patient's condition is either stable or progressing so slowly that it cannot be determined over a decade. If the nerves in 2011 appear clearly worse than the photographs, then the target pressure should average less than 19 mmHg. Real patients like the hypothetical patient GH do exist; in such patients baseline photographs are very useful.

Patients who have early or moderate perimetric disease often show convincing changes in their fields before clear progressive changes in the nerves are evident. However, not all patients can perform good field tests, and media opacities may develop that affect the field but do not preclude examination of the nerve. Photographs of the nerves are of little value when there is very advanced cupping.

Disc hemorrhages. The observation of a splinter hemorrhage along the disc margin on a routine disc examination may mean that a patient's condition is unstable.[1,2] If a disc hemorrhage is noted, perform a visual field examination and an OCT-RNFL analysis within the next 1 to 3 months, depending on the severity of the patient's disease. If there is visual field worsening or RNFL thinning ≥ 5 microns in the area corresponding to the hemorrhage, this constitutes evidence of glaucomatous progression, since the two findings support one another. If the field or OCT-RNFL shows no change, repeat the tests in 3 to 6 months, depending on the severity of the disease. In patients with severely constricted visual fields, a disc hemorrhage itself is considered evidence of glaucomatous progression.

OCT-RNFL changes. In patients with pre-perimetric glaucoma, progressive thinning of the RNFL in the absence of other pathologies may indicate glaucomatous progression. Similarly, in a glaucoma suspect without a visual field defect (with or without high pressure), progressive RNFL thinning not attributed to other causes may indicate conversion to manifest glaucoma (Chapter 3). In most spectral-domain OCT-RNFL analyses, between-visit variability of mean circumpapillary RNFL thickness is probably higher in early compared to moderate or severe glaucoma, when the RNFL may be near depletion.* The value of OCT-RNFL analysis in individuals with moderate to severe field loss depends on the degree of RNFL loss. If the RNFL is very thin, OCT may be useless in detecting progressive damage. We consider glaucoma progression to have occurred if either of the following is present (Chart 5-1):

- Confirmed thinning of mean RNFL thickness ≥ 10 microns.
- Confirmed thinning of mean RNFL thickness ≥ 5 microns with corresponding visual field changes and/or disc hemorrhage.

When glaucoma is severe and the RNFL is depleted, any further glaucomatous loss no longer results in detectable corresponding RNFL changes.[5] Thus, when the average RNFL thickness is below 60 microns and/or the mean visual field deviation is worse than -15 dB, the presence of progressive thinning on OCT-RNFL analysis may indicate glaucoma progression, but the absence of progressive thinning does not always indicate stability.

---

* The "tolerance limit," or change attributed to normal test-retest variability in $\leq 5\%$ of patients, is 3.89 microns in patients with moderate/severe glaucoma,[3] while the average intervisit variability can be as much as 4.85 microns in normal eyes.[4]

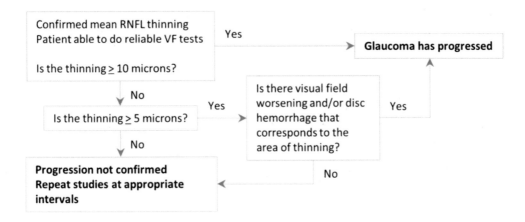

CHART 5-1. Detecting glaucoma progression using OCT-RNFL as a guide in a patient able to perform reliable visual fields. For patients unable to perform reliable visual fields, see discussion on page 121-124. Key – RNFL (retinal nerve fiber layer, as measured by optical coherence tomography).

Visual field as a guide. The ability to recognize marginal progression depends on the quality of the baseline fields as well as on the degree of initial visual field loss. The more damaged a portion of the field, the more it may vary both on repeat measure and from day to day, and thus the more difficult it is to recognize additional deterioration. Therefore on follow-up examinations, it should be determined if the field shows change beyond the expected variation and, if it does, whether the change is related to progressive glaucomatous damage or to some other cause. The only clear standard for diagnosing progressive glaucomatous damage on automated static threshold perimetry is that a change should be confirmed on a repeat examination, especially if the field change is the only sign that indicates worsening. If the field change is confirmed by another finding, for example, a corresponding disc hemorrhage, focal thinning on OCT-RNFL analysis, a distinctly uncontrolled pressure, or a cup that has clearly enlarged, it may be better to repeat the field as a new baseline after taking the next appropriate management step. Confirmation of a field change is important because whatever reasonable criteria are used to recognize marginal progression, a patient whose condition is stable will meet the criteria occasionally because of the variability in field testing. Aggressive treatment in a patient whose disease is stable is unwarranted if the clinician happens to test the field on a day when the patient's visual sensitivity was decreased by something other than progressive glaucoma. Visual fields may deteriorate in one or more of three main ways:

- A new defect may develop in a previously normal area.
- A preexisting defect may deepen and/or expand.
- The entire field may develop decreased sensitivity.

The two fundamental rules for the interpretation of a series of visual fields are first, to compare each individual follow-up field, as it is obtained, to the baseline fields and second, to study the entire series of fields since diagnosis to see if there is any feature that shows a steady decline beyond any field-to-field variability. A statistical program facilitates each approach, but both may be done without one. The following discussion deals with the use of the STATPAC and Guided Progression Analysis (GPA) programs.

Comparison of an individual field to the field baseline. GPA uses the first two reliable visual fields as a baseline unless there is a marked learning effect in which case it will discard the first field. Subsequent fields are compared to the baseline and the Visual Field Index of all fields is displayed. If progression is possible or likely, an alert appears.

If the GPA is not available, choose the most reliable of the baseline fields for pointwise comparison. Each follow-up field should be compared to the baseline field and not to interim fields to avoid missing gradual worsening. Glaucomatous changes between each field in a series may be small enough such that progression is missed unless the most recent field is compared to the baseline.

In general, more stringent criteria are required to detect progression of an expanding or deepening defect than a new onset defect due to the inherent higher variability within preexisting visual field defects. HAP2 criteria part III provides guidelines for detecting visual field changes (page 106). A step-wise approach is outlined on the next page.

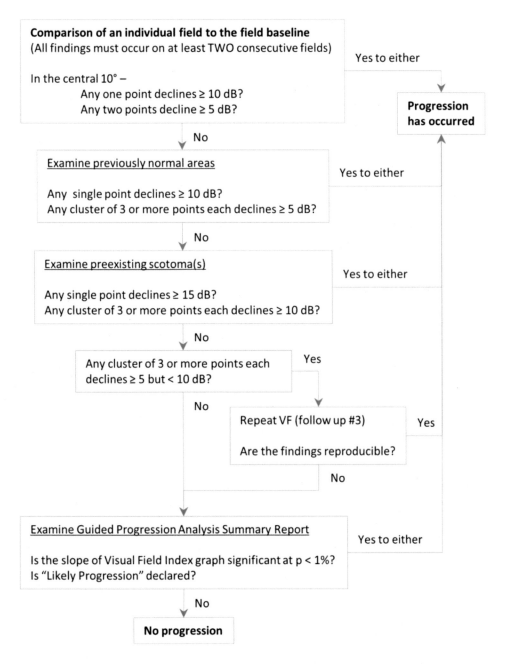

CHART 5-2. A step-wise approach to comparing an individual field to the field baseline based on HAP2 criteria part III (next page).

HAP2 Criteria, Part III
Criteria for Visual Field Progression

In previously normal areas, any of the following on at least TWO consecutive fields:

- A single point that declines ≥ 10 dB in a previously normal area.
- Within the central 10° – two or more points each of which declines ≥ 5 dB compared to baseline.
- Outside the central 10° – a cluster of three or more points each of which declines ≥ 5 dB compared to baseline.

Within a preexisting defect, any of the following on at least TWO consecutive fields:

- A single point that declines ≥ 15 dB within a preexisting defect.
- Within the central 10° – any point that declines ≥ 10 dB.
- Outside the central 10° – a cluster of 3 or more points each of which declines ≥10 dB compared to baseline, or each of which declines ≥ 5 dB on THREE consecutive fields (the confirming points may differ if they are part of a contiguous cluster)

Either of the following on Guided Progression Analysis:

- A slope significant at p < 1% for Visual Field Index graph.
- A "Likely Progression" message on Guided Progression Analysis.

A

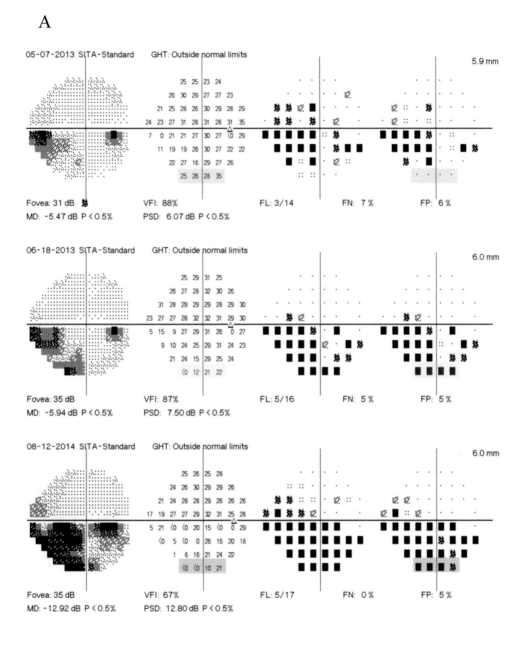

FIG 5-1. Glaucoma progression based on HAP2 criteria part III. New defect in a previously normal area. Previously normal area (*green highlight*) has 4 points each of which declined greater than 5 dB on two consecutive fields (*yellow and red highlights*). The examinations were performed without correction.

B

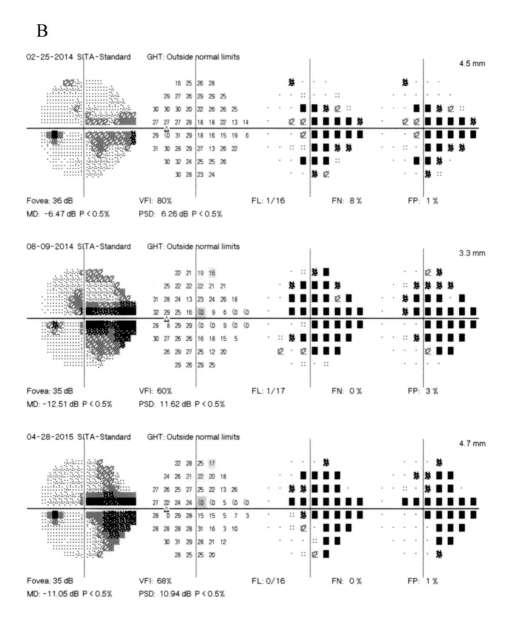

FIG 5-2. Glaucoma progression based on HAP2 criteria part III. Expansion and deepening of a preexisting scotoma into contiguous points. One of the central points (within a preexisting scotoma) is depressed by > 15 dB (*red highlight*), a cluster of 3 points in previously normal area is depressed by > 5 dB (*yellow highlight*), and at least a single point in previously normal area is depressed by > 10 dB (*green highlight*) on repeated exam.

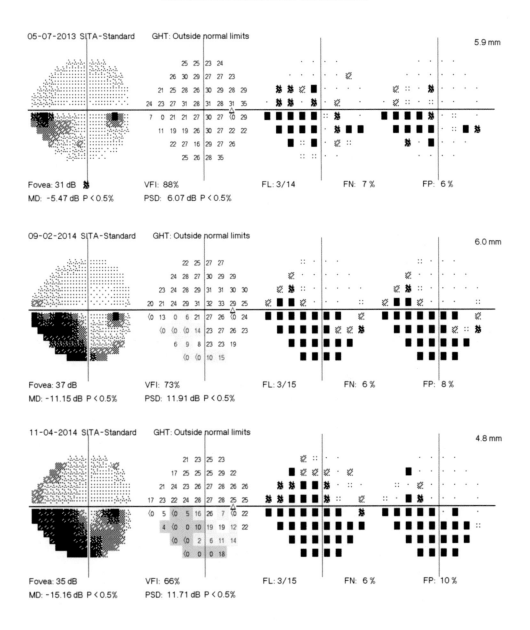

FIG 5-3. Glaucoma progression based on HAP2 part III. Deepening of a preexisting defect. Compared to the baseline from 5/7/2013, the 9/2/14 field shows deepening of the inferior scotoma in several areas by more than 10 dB (*yellow highlight*). An exam on 11/4/14 confirmed the deepening of defect (*red highlight*).

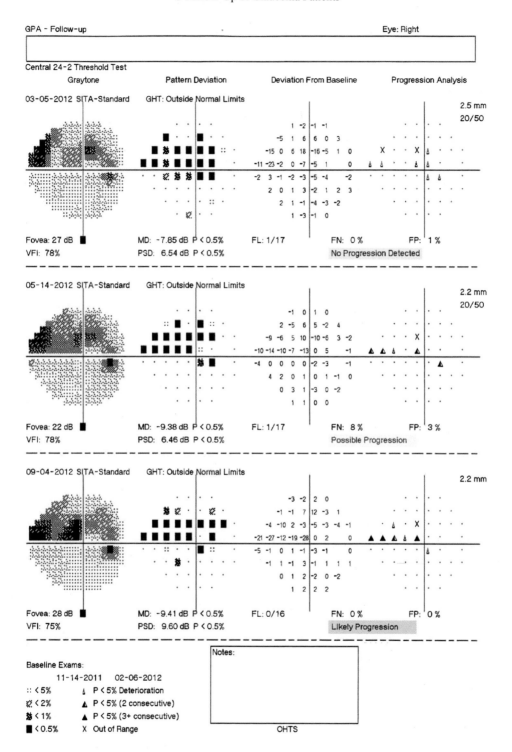

FIG. 5-4. Glaucoma progression based on HAP2 part III. Progression based on Guided Progression Analysis (GPA). Compared to the baseline, the most recent field exam shows ≥ 3 points which have deteriorated on three or more consecutive follow-up tests (*black triangles*), and the GPA alert shows "Likely Progression" (*red highlight*).

110

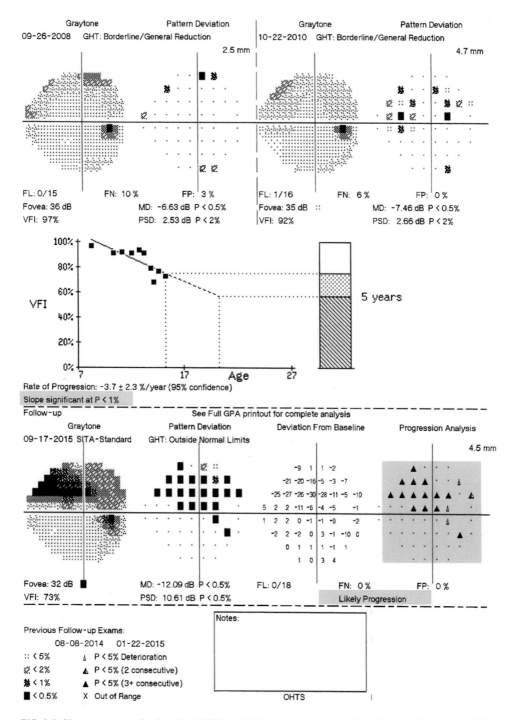

FIG. 5-5. Glaucoma progression based on HAP2 part III. Progression based on Guided Progression Analysis (GPA). The Visual Field Index (VFI) graph shows a negative slope significant at P < 1%. The Glaucoma Change Probability Map shows multiple test points that have deteriorated on three or more consecutive follow-up exams (*black triangles*), and the GPA alert displays "Likely Progression" (*red highlights*). This young patient required multiple surgeries to control his glaucoma.

The limitations of statistical programs and visual fields. Statistical programs provide probabilities, but they do not practice medicine. They do not determine if a change is a transient physiologic one or a permanent pathologic change. They do not determine if a change is related to glaucoma or to a retinal vascular occlusion, tumor, or stroke. The field needs to be interpreted in light of the entire clinical picture.

Modifying the Target Pressure

If a person with glaucoma tolerates his or her treatment, if the pressure stays at or below the target, and if the nerve and visual fields remain stable, we do not modify the treatment or ponder whether the target pressure is too low. It is time to reassess the patient's management when the patient develops intolerance to medication, when the pressure rises beyond the target, or when the nerve, nerve fiber layer, or field shows progression.

If, after a period of stability, medication intolerance develops or if the pressure rises higher than the target, it may be appropriate to modify the target pressure upward unless a slight change in therapy (such as a substitution of another medication in the same class) achieves the original target pressure. The longer the patient has been followed without progression before developing medication intolerance or exceeding the target pressure, the more confident the clinician can be that the pressure maintained during that interval was indeed low enough, and that a somewhat higher IOP might be adequate. In general, if the patient's condition has been stable for at least two years, we are willing to reset the target pressure up to 4 mmHg higher in a patient with early to moderate disease and up to 2 mmHg above the initial target in a patient with severe disease. If the target is reset upward, then the patient should be followed up closely for a time to determine stability. A patient with mild disease should have a visual field and an OCT-RNFL test every 6 months for 1 year; a patient with moderate disease every 6 months for 2 years, and a patient with severe disease every 3 to 4 months for a year and then every 6 months for another year. For moderate and severe disease, OCT should be repeated yearly if the mean RNFL thickness is ≥ 60 microns.

If the glaucomatous damage progresses, the target pressure should usually be revised downward. Reassess the risk/benefit ratio of more aggressive treatment given the patient's duration and degree of disease before pursuing aggressive treatment. For example, a patient with mild or moderate disease who is 70 years old and whose condition worsens slightly over a decade may be at less visual risk from IOP than he or she would be from filtration surgery.

Modifying Treatment

Medication Intolerance

A common circumstance that requires a change in management is the development of intolerance to medication that was originally tolerated. Sometimes an alternate medication or laser trabeculoplasty achieves the target pressure easily. However, if the pressure rises above the target pressure, then the target should be reevaluated as described above.

Local intolerance. Drops may cause contact dermatitis of the eyelids and an associated conjunctival allergic reaction, with itching as a prominent symptom. Chronic reactive hyperemia or follicular conjunctivitis on a nonallergic basis may also occur, as may a pemphigoid type of conjunctival scarring. Whatever the basis, if symptomatic cutaneous or conjunctival reaction develops, discontinue the medication. Sometimes a preservative-free formulation of the medication can be used, but it is usually more expeditious to use another therapy. If the conjunctival reaction could have represented viral or bacterial conjunctivitis, try the medication again in one eye for a few days after the inflammation resolves.

Beta-blocker intolerance. If either respiratory or cardiac disease develops that could be related to beta-blockade, discontinue the beta-blocker while determining if the drug is indeed contributing to the problem. Tolerated beta-blocker treatment does not usually become intolerable suddenly in the absence of another process. Thus a patient who notes a sudden change in symptomatology should have a prompt evaluation by his or her general medical physician. Individuals who become intolerant to betaxolol cannot use any other beta-blocker. Those who develop respiratory intolerance to a nonselective beta-blocker may tolerate betaxolol. Do not use betaxolol in patients who develop cardiac failure with nonselective blockers.

Prostaglandin analog intolerance. Intolerance to prostaglandin analogs is commonly due to symptoms of irritation and burning and less commonly due to hyperpigmentation of the skin and/or iris, lash growth, and prostaglandin-associated periorbitopathy. Even mild hyperpigmentation, lash growth, or orbital contour changes can be noticeable and cosmetically undesirable if unilateral. Pigment changes and orbital fat redistribution may be irreversible. If cosmetic changes are due to unilateral usage, some patients will accept bilateral application to minimize asymmetry in appearance. If the pressure is well-controlled on a benzalkonium chloride-containing prostaglandin analog and the main cause of intolerability is irritation, a short trial with a prostaglandin analog that either uses an alternative preservative or is preservative-free will sort out whether the medication or the preservative is to blame. Occasionally, a patient may become intolerant to one particular prostaglandin analog but do well with another.

Alpha-agonist intolerance. Brimonidine causes localized allergic reaction with itching and redness in some patients. It can also result in dry mouth, somnolence or fatigue. A monocular, once daily trial may help determine whether the patient is susceptible to these side effects before using the full dose. If the patient reports side effects, choose another medication. In some patients apraclonidine may be a tolerable substitute as it does not cross the blood-brain barrier as readily, although it is also less effective.

Systemic carbonic anhydrase inhibitor intolerance. Chronic use of systemic carbonic anhydrase inhibitors is rare unless patients both have significant disease and fail to achieve control on other treatment. Symptomatic side effects usually occur shortly after the medication is started. However, lethargy and depression may be insidious, either not recognized at first or not attributed to the drug until some later time. Late intolerance may also arise because the patient grows tired of the side effects of the pills. Either way, relative intolerance of systemic carbonic anhydrase inhibitors usually involves choosing to live with the side effects, having a higher than desired pressure, or having glaucoma surgery. A reasonable course in a patient with relative intolerance is to stop the carbonic anhydrase inhibitor, perform incisional surgery in one eye, and observe the other eye. If the operated eye does well, surgery on the second eye can be done. If the surgery does not go well on the first eye, either because of poor pressure control or visually significant side effects, and if the unoperated eye worsens, the clinician and the patient may elect to resume the systemic carbonic anhydrase inhibitor and tolerate the side effects rather than do surgery on the second eye.

Pressure Increase

Pressure increase includes a variety of situations, most of which fall into one of three groups: a sudden marked increase in IOP compared to previous readings, a mild to moderate change in pressure that results in pressure above the target, or a gradual increase in IOP over several visits regardless of whether the target pressure is passed. In each case, examine the eye for some obvious cause such as inflammation and perform gonioscopy to rule out the development of angle closure, neovascularization of the angle, or elevated episcleral venous pressure. If angle closure is found, it is usually secondary to pupillary block and an iridotomy is the appropriate treatment. If no obvious cause is found, then the likely explanations and management depend on the circumstances of presentation.

Sudden dramatic increase in pressure. Patients with chronic glaucoma rarely have rapid changes in their condition. If a pressure reading is markedly elevated compared to previous readings, the three most common explanations (other than angle closure) in our experience are that:

1. The patient failed to use his or her medication;
2. The patient has pseudoexfoliation syndrome;
3. The patient is under unusual major stress (a child using drugs has been incarcerated, a spouse has died, a bitter divorce has gone to court, etc.).

The latter cause (acute stress) is one that we have noted frequently enough to accept as a valid reason for deviation from pressure control.

If the patient missed a dose of medication but his or her condition is otherwise stable and the patient denies frequent noncompliance, recheck the pressure after the person uses his or her medication. If the patient is known to have or found to have pseudoexfoliation and a second IOP determination confirms the pressure rise, proceed with additional treatment following the guidelines for established glaucoma. Patients in this situation may require laser treatment or incisional surgery if the pressure is to be kept at or below the set target. If the patient is undergoing unusual stress and the examination does not reveal any other explanation, then the patient should return soon and the pressure should be rechecked. If the pressure is so high or the eye is so damaged that it requires prompt treatment, proceed with additional treatment as described in Chapter 4. Otherwise, it is often acceptable to allow the stress and the pressure to subside rather than to modify the patient's regimen. Sometimes the pressure rises suddenly and no explanation is found. In such cases, progress with additional treatment as described in Chapter 4.

Mild to moderate change in pressure that increases pressure above the target. Consider, for example, a pressure rise of 5 mmHg that raises the pressure 2 mmHg above the target in a person without progressive nerve or field damage. If the higher IOP is still below the initial untreated pressure and if the patient's condition has been stable for at least a year, it may be appropriate to modify the target pressure as previously discussed. If the patient has not been followed up long enough to determine stability, we recommend rechecking the pressure on a different day before changing the treatment course. For patients with mild disease, recheck the pressure within 2 months. For patients with moderate disease, recheck within 1 month, and recheck patients with severe disease within 2 weeks. If the pressure remains elevated beyond the target pressure on repeat pressure checking, proceed as described in Chapter 4.

Gradual rise in pressure over time. If gonioscopy fails to show progressive angle closure, then the usual explanation for this finding is that either the medications are gradually losing their effectiveness or that the underlying resistance to aqueous humor outflow is rising. Provided the pressure remains below the target and the field and OCT-RNFL remain stable, observe the patient without changing treatment. If the pressure rises above the target, reevaluate the target as described above. Then, if indicated, proceed with additional treatment as described in Chapter 4.

Worsening Visual Fields, Disc, or Retinal Nerve Fiber Layers

Most patients who show worsening of their fields or whose nerves and retinal nerve fiber layers appear to have deteriorated compared to their baseline studies (either photos or OCT-RNFL analyses) fit into one of three general classes:

1. Rapid worsening despite achievement and maintenance of the target pressure;
2. Rapid worsening associated with failure to achieve the desired target pressure;
3. Gradual worsening with or without achievement of the target pressure.

Unless the worsening is part of a generally uncontrolled situation, a repeat field test or repeat optic nerve studies (photo and/or OCT-RNFL analysis) should confirm the worsening before management is changed.

Rapid worsening despite achievement and maintenance of target pressure –

Probable causes. Glaucoma may progress rapidly, but unless the pressure is substantially above the threshold for damage, it usually progresses in small steps. When a patient's condition is worsening rapidly despite achievement of the desired pressure, there are four major possibilities to consider:

1. The patient has a very low threshold for damage because of many non-pressure risk factors.
2. The patient does not take his or her medicine between visits.
3. The pressure fluctuates widely, and thus for part of the time, the target pressure has not been achieved.
4. Something other than or in addition to glaucoma is causing the field loss.

Although the explanation often is that the patient is not using medication properly, the possibility that additional visual loss is not related to glaucoma demands the most immediate attention. The list of urgent concerns includes – but is not limited to – tumor, anterior ischemic optic neuropathy, retinal vascular occlusion, and giant cell arteritis. If the patient has had a clearly stable course for a period of time and then shows clear deterioration while maintaining target pressure, a nonglaucomatous cause must be suspected. Late deterioration can occur if the patient's general health declines and the optic nerve becomes more susceptible to pressure, but such rapid change occurs rarely.

Diagnostic approach. Reexamine the patient. Take a careful history. This should include questions about medication compliance. Not everyone will admit to failure to use medications, but some patients will. Ask about any other symptoms that the patient may have that suggest either vascular events or mass lesions. Check the acuity and note if it is falling. Check color vision. In some people it is appropriate to use an Amsler grid to look for central scotomas. Repeat gonioscopy to check for previously missed angle closure that could be raising the pressure intermittently. Look carefully at the nerve and determine if it is consistent with the visual field and/or OCT-RNFL changes. In particular, look for shunt vessels and pallor out of proportion to cupping each of which suggests a nonglaucomatous optic neuropathy. Examine the rest of the fundus for conditions such as vascular narrowing consistent with a branch vascular occlusion.

Study the visual field carefully and determine if it is unusual for glaucoma. Is there a central scotoma or a homonymous defect that might be more consistent with a pathologic condition in the orbit or brain? Did a major field defect, such as a total hemifield loss or a dense nerve fiber bundle defect, appear from one field to the next, as might occur in a person with acute anterior ischemic optic neuropathy? If the field is atypical in any manner, proceed further. This may involve orbital echography and neuroimaging studies. Consultation with a neurologist or neuro-ophthalmologist is particularly helpful in planning an appropriate diagnostic approach in this situation. Check the pressure at different times of the day, especially if the patient had wide pressure fluctuations before treatment.

If all findings seem consistent with chronic glaucoma, then assume that the worsening is pressure related.

Therapeutic approach. Treat any nonglaucomatous conditions identified. If the worsening is determined to be glaucomatous, reset a target pressure goal 30% lower than the initial target. When this situation arises we have generally elected to perform filtration surgery, at least in one eye, because filtration surgery is the best means to achieve a consistently very low pressure. The risks of surgery to a person whose condition is deteriorating rapidly have generally seemed reasonable.

Rapid worsening associated with failure to achieve the desired target pressure. Some patients will have higher than desired pressures during follow-up. The initial target pressure is only an estimate, and if easy measures reduce the pressure to a level near the target, we may accept a higher than desired pressure for a while and evaluate the rate of further damage. Often the decision to accept a pressure above the target is made when the next treatment option is either a systemic carbonic anhydrase inhibitor or incisional surgery. Of course, these patients' conditions can worsen from causes other than glaucoma, and we recommend that the patient be examined carefully to confirm that any change is glaucomatous in nature. However, it is not surprising if progressive damage develops in a patient with inadequately lowered IOP. When a patient's condition is rapidly worsening because of glaucoma, we perform aggressive incisional surgery to achieve prompt pressure control. It is usually futile to encourage compliance or try to change medications when the situation is clearly uncontrolled.

Gradual worsening regardless of whether the target pressure has been achieved. Over the years, many patients with glaucoma lose some of their retinal ganglion cells and visual field. Some will have "well-controlled" pressures, and some will have less than the desired pressure lowering. Worsening usually signals that there should be a change in management. The extent of change in the target pressure and management do not depend on the fact that progression has occurred, but on how serious the damage was initially and the rate of progression on the treatment used to date. Once progression has occurred, the time period over which the progression occurred lends clues to the rate of change. The steps in this situation are similar to those involved in instituting treatment.

Diagnostic approach. Determine the rate of change. The pace at which the condition is worsening helps in deciding how aggressive treatment should be to obtain an even lower pressure. If a 79-year-old person had only mild or moderate field loss initially and has had a mild enlargement of a scotoma over the past 10 years, it is reasonable not to change management unless the damage accelerates. The same change in a 45-year-old patient almost always warrants more aggressive treatment.

Try to determine if the patient is compliant with treatment. If poor compliance is established, it may be best to try a treatment, such as laser or incisional surgery, which does not require chronic medication use.

Therapeutic approach. Reset the target pressure. The degree of initial damage and rate of further change help to determine how much lower to aim in pressure control. For example, clear-cut change may be noted over 3 years or 15 years, and the two situations are treated differently. The more rapid the change, the greater should be the additional lowering. When resetting the target pressure, we recommend trying to achieve about a 25% further reduction in average pressure (15% for progression that occurs over > 5 years, and 35% for progression that occurs over < 2 years), compared to the average pressures of the patient during the period of change.

Treat to achieve the new target pressure. If the rate of progression is a serious threat in a given patient, consider bleb-forming incisional surgery if additional medical therapy or non-bleb forming surgeries are unlikely to have a prompt, dramatic effect.

Establish a new baseline and start a new follow-up schedule. If progression was determined by visual field criteria, the two fields that showed progression may serve as a baseline. However, if a miotic was added or if surgery was performed, it is best to obtain new fields promptly. In most cases, the clinician should obtain new optic nerve studies. In the future, this new baseline will be used for comparison, and all the provisos about the ability to determine change apply to the new baseline.[*]

The Patient with Progressive Glaucoma and Low Baseline IOP

Progression of disease despite medical and/or laser therapy does not mean that pressure is the sole causative factor, but it does indicate that a person's condition is at very high risk to continue to worsen. The lower the pretreatment IOP, the higher the probability that surgery will be required to achieve the initial target IOP. When a patient with low baseline IOP has progressive damage, comparing the course of the two eyes may be helpful. We usually operate on at least one eye to lower the pressure. Table 5-3 (page 120) outlines a management plan to follow if progression occurs.

One eye had surgery and achieved a substantially lower pressure. If a patient's condition shows convincing progression, confirmed on repeat examination, then the treatment should be adjusted accordingly.

- If the operated eye is stable while the fellow eye progressed, then operate on the fellow eye to achieve at least the IOP of the previously operated eye. Continue to follow up with the patient.
- If both eyes progressed but the operated eye progressed less than the unoperated eye, then operate on the fellow eye and augment medical therapy in both eyes with a target IOP 20% lower than the mean IOP already achieved by surgery in the previously operated eye.

---

[*]The clinician can manually select the new baseline fields for Guided Progression Analysis.[6]

- If the unoperated eye has fared better than the operated eye, reevaluate the patient for nonglaucomatous causes of visual loss.
- If a operated eye has no glaucomatous progression but loses vision related to surgery, for example, corneal edema or hypotony maculopathy, while the fellow eye develops progressive glaucomatous damage, treat the previously unoperated eye up to the point at which the complications occurred, in the hope that with submaximal treatment the initially unoperated eye fares better overall than the other eye. This can be a difficult decision at times.

Neither eye had surgery, both eyes progressing –

- If the pressures in the two eyes are symmetric, advance therapy in both eyes but perform surgery only on the worse-seeing eye to achieve a new target IOP of 20% lowering of the mean IOP during progression. Continue to observe the patient's other eye without surgery and decide whether to operate depending on the course in the operated eye.
- If the pressures are consistently asymmetric, and if the eye with the higher IOP has progressed more than the other eye, this supports a pressure-related element to the damage. Advance therapy in both eyes but operate only on the eye with higher IOP to achieve a target that is 20% lower than the average IOP during progression. Continue to observe the condition of both eyes. Proceed with surgery in the unoperated eye after sufficient time has elapsed to be confident of a favorable course in the first eye.
- If the pressures are consistently asymmetric, and if the eye with the higher IOP has fared better than the other eye, operate on the eye with the lower IOP to achieve a 20% lowering of average IOP. Continue to observe the other eye without surgery. Pressure may be a factor in this situation, but the evidence is less compelling than if the eye with the higher pressure worsened.

Both eyes had surgery and achieved substantially lower pressures –

- If the pressures in the two eyes are symmetric and one or both are worse, commit to achieving an additional 20% lowering of IOP in the worse-seeing eye using whatever means necessary. Continue to observe the other eye and decide whether to augment treatment depending on the course in the more aggressively treated eye.
- If the pressures are consistently asymmetric, and if the eye with the higher IOP is worse than the other eye, treat both eyes with a target of 20% additional lowering of IOP. If additional surgery is required, do it in only one eye initially. Proceed with the other eye depending on the course in the first eye.
- If the pressures are consistently asymmetric, and if the eye with the higher IOP has fared better than the fellow eye, commit to achieving a 20% additional lowering of IOP in the worse eye using whatever means necessary. Continue to observe the other eye without advancing treatment. This course commits one eye to each course of treatment, although the initial response does not support a large component of pressure-related damage.

The management of glaucoma with low baseline IOP is frustrating for the patient and for the doctor. We recommend explaining to the patient – early, emphatically, and repeatedly – that the best course is not known and that the purpose of treatment is to provide the best chance possible of having appropriate treatment in at least one eye.

TABLE 5-3. Management of progressive glaucoma with low baseline IOP.

Initial approach	Outcome	Suggested modification
One eye had surgery	Operated eye stable, unoperated eye progressed	Operate on the unoperated eye
	Both eyes progressed, but operated eye progressed less	Operate on the unoperated eye and augment medical therapy in both eyes with a new target of 20% lower than the first operated eye's mean IOP during progression
	Operated eye progressed; unoperated eye stable	Evaluate the patient for nonglaucomatous causes of field loss
	Operated eye has no progression but loses vision related to surgery; fellow eye progressed	Treat the unoperated eye up to the point at which the surgical complications in the other eye occurred
Neither eye had surgery, both eyes progressing	IOP symmetric	Operate on the worse-seeing eye to achieve a target of at least 20% lowering of the mean IOP during progression; manage the other eye medically pending assessment of result of surgery
	IOP asymmetric, higher IOP eye has progressed more	Operate on the eye with higher IOP for a target of 20% lower than the mean IOP of other eye during progression; observe the fellow eye pending assessment of result of surgery
	IOP asymmetric, higher IOP eye has progressed less	Operate on the eye with lower IOP for a target of at least a 20% lowering of IOP; observe the fellow eye pending assessment of result of surgery
Both eyes had surgery and achieved a substantial lowering of IOP, both eyes progressing	IOP symmetric	Commit the worse-seeing eye to an additional 20% lowering of IOP; do not operate on the fellow eye pending assessment of the more-treated eye
	IOP asymmetric, higher IOP eye has progressed more	Augment medical therapy to both eyes with a target 20% lower than the IOP in the lower IOP eye; if surgery is needed, operate on the worse-seeing eye only pending assessment of result of surgery
	IOP asymmetric, higher IOP eye has progressed less	Commit the worse-seeing eye to a trial of lowering IOP maximally; observe the fellow eye

Following Up on Treatment Variations

In Chapter 4 we outlined our initial approach to three groups of patients who did not fit easily into the routine management scheme for chronic glaucoma: those who cannot do reliable fields, those whose fundi cannot be seen, and those with advanced disease when first seen. For each group, follow-up care presents the expected difficulties.

The Patient Who Cannot Do Reliable Fields

The obvious problem in following individuals who cannot perform reliable fields is that it may take a large increment of damage to be recognizable. The greater the degree of initial damage, the greater a problem this presents. The difficulty in following the rate of change in these patients highlights the value of field examinations. As with patients with routine chronic glaucoma, the frequency of follow-up depends on the degree of damage and the extent to which the pressure is lowered. In general, if the nerve has only mild damage and is easily examined, it is possible to recognize mild to moderate progression if the patient has good, high-resolution stereoscopic baseline photographs and a good OCT-RNFL baseline.

Role of OCT-RNFL analyses. In the absence of useful fields, serial OCT-RNFL analyses, if reproducible with good quality, can be used to detect progression. We make the following assumptions –

1. Progressive RNFL thinning occurs with increasing glaucoma severity.
2. An abnormal (thinner) RNFL may demonstrate less between-visit variability than a normal (thicker) RNFL.
3. The more severe the glaucoma, the greater the potential functional loss with each increment of loss of RNFL thickness.

Hence, for patients who cannot do reliable fields, we accept a confirmed mean RNFL thinning of 8 microns or more as evidence of progression in those categorized as early glaucoma (Table 4-1, page 91) and thinning of 4 microns or more as progression in those categorized as moderate or severe glaucoma. This is a more stringent criterion than in patients able to do reliable fields (10 microns if follow-up fields remain normal, 5 microns if accompanied by any new field defect or disc hemorrhages). In a patient with a depleted or nearly-depleted RNFL (average less than 60 microns), stable OCT-RNFL analyses do not rule out progression. [5]

Once it is known that deterioration is not rapid in a patient with early or moderate glaucoma, follow-up may be similar to patients who can perform reliable fields. In more advanced cases, successive nerve and RNFL evaluation is less valuable, and strict pressure control and frequent visits will be necessary. Sometimes a patient with serious visual loss can accurately describe visual fluctuations and can report meaningfully that his or her vision is or is not generally stable. In such cases, a subjective sense of deteriorating vision (especially dimming) may be the prime guide to more aggressive therapy.

We suggest the following as examples of follow-up schedules. On every visit the clinician should examine the optic disc, particularly to detect disc hemorrhages; gonioscopy should be performed every 1-2 years in phakic patients.

Case IJ – easily controlled early glaucoma. A 60-year-old asymptomatic woman is first seen with an IOP of 32 mmHg and a nerve with cup/disc ratio of 0.5 with neural rim tissue of good color without notches or hemorrhages. Baseline examinations include pressure measurements averaging 30 mmHg (range, 27 to 33 mmHg) and excellent-quality optic nerve photographs. OCT-RNFL analysis shows normal overall thickness (green) that has thinned by 11-13 microns compared to a study performed elsewhere 4 years ago. The contour shows superior and inferior thinning. Despite education and multiple attempts, the patient cannot perform reliable visual fields. This patient, with normal average RNFL thickness but abnormal RNFL contour, is thought to have early glaucoma (Table 4-1, page 91). The initial target pressure is 25% lowering of pre-treatment pressure, or a target of 23 mmHg. Treatment with a beta-blocker results in a pressure of 21 mmHg after 1 month. This initial evaluation took approximately 9 weeks.

- When should this patient be reexamined?
- What should be tested on follow-up?

Over time, it will be important to determine if the optic nerve is developing progressive damage, but initially the focus is on the pressure. Once the initial target pressure is achieved, it is reasonable to examine this patient in a month or so to check the pressure. If it remains low, reexamine the patient again in 2 or 3 months and examine the optic nerve. If the nerve is stable and the pressure remains within the target, see the patient again in 3 months (6 months into follow-up) to check the pressure, dilate the patient's pupils for funduscopy, and repeat the OCT-RNFL analysis. A stable OCT-RNFL analysis at this point may or may not suggest long-term stability, but progressive thinning of 8 microns or more indicates poor control. In another 3 months, check the pressure, and 3 months thereafter (now 12 months into follow-up), test the pressure, repeat gonioscopy, dilate the patient's pupils to examine the disc and fundus, and repeat the OCT-RNFL analysis. Check the IOP and nerve every 6 months, and repeat the OCT-RNFL and disc photos 2 years into follow-up. If the patient's condition appears to be stable, and if the pressure remains within the target range, then decrease the frequency of pressure and nerve examinations to every 9 months for 2 or 3 more years; repeat the OCT-RNFL analysis at every visit; perform gonioscopy, dilated fundus exam and obtain disc photos every other visit. If the OCT-RNFL and photos show stability through 5 years into follow-up, follow the patient yearly with dilated fundus exam, and OCT-RNFL. Obtain photographs at least every 2 years and always compare the new photographs to the initial photographs. OCT technology can change and analyses performed by different software may be difficult to compare, but a high-quality disc photograph can be used for comparison whether presented digitally, on film, or on paper (Table 5-2).

If on any of the repeat examinations, the OCT-RNFL or optic nerve photos document progression, then reset the target pressure at least 20% lower than the initial target and treat the patient for moderate disease.

Case KL – probably controlled moderate glaucoma. A 59-year-old man with excellent vision has untreated pressures that average 28 mmHg (range, 24 to 32 mmHg). His cup/disc ratio is 0.7 with a notch inferotemporally in both optic nerves, and OCT-RNFL analysis shows average thickness between the 1st and 5th percentile (yellow) with focal thinning of several inferotemporal clock hours below the 1st percentile (red). Despite extensive patient education, fields are totally unreliable. He is thought to have moderate glaucoma (Table 4-1, page 91) and an initial target pressure is set at 17 mmHg. Beta-blocker use is contraindicated because of severe asthma. Treatment with a prostaglandin analog results in pressures of 22 mmHg. A trial of brimonidine produces intolerable symptoms. Addition of topical carbonic anhydrase inhibitor lowers the pressure to 17 mmHg. The patient is maintained on both a prostaglandin analog and a topical carbonic anhydrase inhibitor. The initial evaluation spanned 3 months and 5 visits.

- When should this patient be reexamined?
- What should be tested on follow-up?

This patient has a distinctly abnormal optic nerve that makes the diagnosis of glaucoma highly likely, but he is very unlikely to show measurable optic nerve changes within only a few months. Recheck the pressure and do an undilated disc exam in about a month and again about two months later (3 months into follow-up). If the pressure is stable, recheck the pressure, dilate the patient's pupils to examine the nerve, and repeat the OCT-RNFL analysis in 3 more months (6 months into follow-up). Test the pressure in 3 more months, and repeat tonometry, gonioscopy, dilated funduscopy and OCT-RNFL analysis in 3 more months (now 12 months into follow-up). If stable, lengthen the follow-up intervals to every 4 months and perform a disc examination and an OCT-RNFL analysis through a dilated pupil at every visit for another year. If stable at 2 years into follow-up, lengthen the follow-up intervals to 6 months. Perform gonioscopy and repeat the nerve photographs and compare them to initial photographs every other visit. If stable through the next 3 years, lengthen the follow-up intervals to 9-12 months (Table 5-2). Repeat OCT-RNFL analysis every visit and gonioscopy every 1-2 years. If the pressure rises above the target, treat as described above.

If the patient's nerves or RNFL show progressive damage (thinning of 4 microns or more) compared to baseline, or if serial photographs document progression, reset the pressure level 25% below the level at which the progression occurred and treat on the frequency schedule for severe glaucoma. Proceed with laser and incisional surgery if needed to achieve the target.

Case MN – marginally controlled severe glaucoma. A 64-year-old man has pressures averaging 26 mmHg (range, 23 to 29 mmHg), with a cup/disc ratio of 0.85 and loss of the inferotemporal rim in both eyes. The OCT-RNFL analysis shows average thickness below the 1st percentile (65 microns, red) with significant thinning in the superior and inferior quadrants (red). The patient cannot perform reliable fields. Baseline photographs are of good quality. This patient with abnormal mean RNFL thickness and contour is assumed to have severe glaucoma (Table 4-1). The target pressure is set at 14 mmHg. With use of a nonselective beta-blocker, the pressure falls to 19 mmHg one week later, and remains 19 mmHg after six weeks. With the addition of a topical carbonic anhydrase inhibitor, IOP falls to 16 mmHg. A laser trabeculoplasty in one eye in conjunction with medication achieves a pressure of 14 mmHg a month after completion of the treatment; laser surgery is performed in the fellow eye. He is maintained on 2 agents. Initial treatment occurs over about 4 months, after which the nerve appears stable on dilated examination with stable OCT-RNFL thickness.

- When should this patient be reexamined?
- What should be tested on follow-up?

This patient has severe disease and a low target pressure, which has been achieved. Examine the patient in one month to determine whether the pressure remains low. If the pressure is still controlled, recheck the pressure in another 2 months. If the patient's condition seems stable, check the pressure every 2-3 months for 24 months. Examine the nerve after the patient's pupils are dilated every 6 months, and obtain an OCT-RNFL analysis and compare it to the baseline scan. Thinning of ≥ 4 microns suggests inadequate IOP control, as does the appearance of a disc hemorrhage or decreasing visual acuity not explained by media opacity. In advanced glaucoma with a nearly depleted RNFL, further thinning may be difficult to detect, and the appearance of a disc hemorrhage and/or subjective decline in vision may be the best indicator of poor control. If the patient's condition is stable for 2 years, check the pressures, repeat the OCT-RNFL and examine the patient after the pupils are dilated every 6 months thereafter. Obtain photographs every other year if a change might be recognizable (Table 5-2). If the pressure rises above the target pressure, augment therapy quickly. If additional medical therapy is either not tolerated or not effective, we recommend incisional surgery in one eye, even if progression has not been documented.

If a patient demonstrates progressive nerve damage on OCT-RNFL analysis or has convincing subjective worsening despite a pressure in the low teens, check carefully for the possibility of another process as outlined in Chapter 7. Assuming that none is found, the only treatment is to lower the pressure if at all possible. If the patient has not had filtration surgery, perform filtration surgery with a target pressure of 10 mmHg. We prefer to pursue this course in one eye at a time because the side effects of surgery to maximally lower pressure can be significant. If the target is achieved in one eye without significant side effects, we perform surgery in the other eye.

The Patient Whose Fundus Cannot Be Seen Well Because of Miosis, Cataract, or Other Media Opacity

Provided the visual field on such patients remains stable, management follows the routine guidelines. However, if the field worsens, it is necessary to decide whether the worsening is related to media opacity or to glaucomatous damage. A generalized depression of the field is more likely to be media related than glaucoma related. Deepening of a preexisting scotoma can result from either. If a new scotoma appears in the absence of deepening of preexisting scotomas, the change is probably related to glaucoma in a patient with glaucoma, but it can obviously be caused by any other ocular or nonocular cause of visual field defect. If the media opacity is due to a cataract, we have a low threshold for performing cataract surgery, as it has the benefits of improving vision, improving visualization of the fundus, and, in some cases, lowering the pressure.

The Patient Who Has Advanced Cupping and Visual Field Loss on Initial Examination

Use the schedule in Tables 5-1 and 5-2 (pages 100 and 126) for follow-up of patients with severe glaucoma.

TABLE 5-2. Follow-up schedules for patients who cannot do reliable fields.

Baseline	• At least three IOP measurements at different times of day • At least two threshold visual field examinations (to verify that patient cannot do reliable fields) • Gonioscopy • OCT-RNFL analysis • Disc photographs	Obtain within 2 months
Initial treatment	• Pressure checks and medication adjustment at 1- to 4-week intervals until treatment regimen is established	Complete within 3 months if possible
Follow-up	• See tables below	

Follow-up Phase of Early Glaucomatous Damage Based on OCT-RNFL Analysis

Months	1	3	6	9	12	15	18	21	24	Years 3-5 q9 mos	After year 5 q yr
IOP	x	x	x	x	x	x			x	x	x
Gonioscopy					x				x	Every other visit	x
Disc exam	x	x		x		x				x	
DFE			x		x				x	Every other visit	x
OCT-RNFL			x		x				x	x	x
Disc photos									x	Every other visit	Every 2 years

Follow-up Phase of Moderate Glaucomatous Damage Based on OCT-RNFL Analysis

Months	1	3	6	9	12	16	20	24	Years 3-5 q6 mos	After year 5 q yr
IOP	x	x	x	x	x	x	x	x	x	x
Gonioscopy					x			x	Every other visit	x
Disc exam	x	x		x						
DFE			x		x	x	x	x	x	x
OCT-RNFL			x		x	x	x	x	x	x
Disc photos								x	Every other visit	x*

Follow-up Phase of Severe Glaucomatous Damage Based on OCT-RNFL Analysis

Months	1	3	6	9	12	15	18	21	24	After year 2 q6 mos
IOP	x	x	x	x	x	x	x	x	x	x
Gonioscopy					x				x	Every other visit
Disc exam	x	x		x		x		x		
DFE			x		x		x		x	x
OCT-RNFL			x*		x*		x*		x*	x*
Disc photos									x*	Every 2 years*

*Repeat disc photos and OCT-RNFL only if a change might be recognizable

Key – IOP (intraocular pressure), DFE (dilated fundus exam), OCT-RNFL (optical coherence tomography retinal nerve fiber layer analysis), q6 mos (every 6 months), q 9 mos (every 9 months).

References

1. Daugeliene L, Yamamoto T, Kitazawa Y. Risk factors for visual field damage progression in normal-tension glaucoma eyes. Graefe's Archives for Clinical and Experimental Ophthalmology. 1999;237:105-8.

2. De Moraes CG, Liebmann JM, Park SC, et al. Optic disc progression and rates of visual field change in treated glaucoma. Acta Ophthalmologica. 2013;91:e86-91.

3. Mwanza JC, Chang RT, Budenz DL, Durbin MK, Gendy MG, Shi W, Feuer WJ. Reproducibility of peripapillary retinal nerve fiber layer thickness and optic nerve head parameters measured with cirrus HD-OCT in glaucomatous eyes. Investigative Ophthalmology & Visual Science. 2010 Nov:51(11):5724-30.

4. Ghasia FF, El-Dairi M, Freedman SF, Rajani A, Asrani S. Reproducibility of spectral-domain optical coherence tomography measurements in adult and pediatric glaucoma. Journal of Glaucoma. 2015 Jan;24(1):55-63.

5. Mwanza JC, Budenz DL, Warren JL, Webel AD, Reynolds CE, Barbosa DT, Lin S. Retinal nerve fibre layer thickness floor and corresponding functional loss in glaucoma. British Journal of Ophthalmology. 2015 Jun;99(6):732-7.

6. Heijl A, Patella VM, Bengtsson B. The Field Analyzer Primer, Fourth Edition: Effective Perimetry. Dublin, California: Carl Zeiss Meditec, Inc. 2012. Print.

6 GLAUCOMA SUSPECT I: OCULAR HYPERTENSION

Individuals with open angles and elevated intraocular pressures (IOP) form the largest group of glaucoma suspects. Our recommended regimen for the care of glaucoma suspects with elevated IOP differs little from that for individuals with manifest mild glaucoma. After establishing a baseline, decide whether to treat to lower the IOP by comparing the risk of future glaucoma damage without lowering IOP to the bother, expense, etc. of treatment to lower the pressure. If treatment is chosen, set a target pressure and attempt to achieve it. Finally, regardless of whether the pressure is lowered, follow the patient to determine if he or she is worsening.

Management Steps for Glaucoma Suspects

1. Establish a baseline.
2. Determine the risk of glaucomatous damage.
3. Decide whether to treat the IOP. If treatment is chosen, set a target pressure and attempt to achieve it.
4. Continue to observe all patients for evidence of worsening.

Establishing a Baseline

The initial evaluation for patients with elevated eye pressure is described in Chapter 2. Obtain at least three IOP measurements, preferably at different times and on different days.

Determining the Risk of Glaucomatous Damage

Our recommendations for managing glaucoma suspects with ocular hypertension are based on the following assumptions –

- The pressure at the time a person becomes a glaucoma suspect has probably been present for some years.
- The greater the pressure for any given degree of damage, the higher the threshold for damage in that patient.
- The higher the pressure, the greater the risk of glaucomatous damage.
- The larger the cup, the more likely it is that the cupping is not entirely physiologic.

The observation group of the Ocular Hypertension Treatment Study (OHTS) provided useful information regarding the risk of developing manifest glaucoma damage in patients with IOP between 24 and 32 mmHg.[1] Three risk factors – higher baseline IOP, thinner central corneal thickness (CCT), and increased vertical cup/disc (VCD) ratio – increased the risk of developing glaucoma. As the study concluded prior to the popularization of retinal fiber layer (RNFL) analysis by optical coherence tomography (OCT), we do not know what effect OCT-RNFL measurements would have had on risk calculation. We divide ocular hypertensive glaucoma suspects as follows:

High-risk suspects have a > 20% risk of converting to manifest glaucoma over a 5-year period. Any eye with an IOP > 32 mmHg is at high risk, as are eyes with a CCT ≤ 555 microns and either an IOP > 26 mmHg or a VCD > 0.3. Any eye with defect on OCT-RNFL *or* visual field testing is considered to be at high risk.[*]

Low-risk suspects, on the other hand, have a ≤ 10% risk of conversion to glaucoma over a 5-year period. Anyone who is not a high-risk suspect and has a CCT > 588 microns is low-risk.

Medium-risk suspects do not fulfill either the high-risk or low-risk criteria above, and have a 10 to ≤ 20% risk of converting to manifest glaucoma over a 5-year period.

Deciding Whether to Treat and Planning Follow-Up

Low-risk suspects with ocular hypertension. Low-risk patients may experience worsening of their conditions over time, but such changes are unlikely to happen quickly. We recommend follow-up without treatment. Regular observation should not be considered nontherapy, but rather therapy that is delayed until it is needed. Any progression is likely to appear very slowly, with adequate time to begin active treatment before the damage is severe enough to be symptomatic. Allowing early damage to occur before starting therapy does not make the nerve more susceptible to further harm from pressure.

We think that the benefit of "preventive" treatment in this group is outweighed by the expense, inconvenience, and medical side effects of therapy. We discuss this philosophy with the patient and do rarely treat low-risk patients who request such therapy. These patients are followed semiannually for one year, and yearly afterwards. We generally perform OCT-RNFL analysis and fields yearly. Glaucoma conversion is diagnosed if the patient demonstrates progressive structural and/or functional changes consistent with glaucoma (Chapter 3).

Medium-risk suspects with ocular hypertension. These individuals challenge the doctor to balance the risks and benefits of ocular hypotensive treatment. If a patient's pressures can be lowered, his or her chance of developing glaucomatous damage will decrease. However, not all medium-risk patients need treatment which, once begun, usually continues for life. Although we recommend discussing the advantages and disadvantages of treatment with the patient, few patients in our practice have strong opinions and most want a recommendation. If the fields and OCT-RNFL are reliable and if the nerve is easily examined, we usually follow without treatment. If the patient prefers treatment, we

---

[*] Any eye with both OCT-RNFL *and* corresponding visual field defect in the context of elevated IOP is diagnosed with glaucoma, and the patient is no longer a glaucoma suspect.

recommend a therapeutic trial of topical medicine.

If the fields and OCT-RNFL are not reliable or if it is difficult to examine the nerve, we generally recommend a treatment trial. If the patient tolerates simple medication, which is generally a prostaglandin analog once nightly or beta-blocker once or twice a day, and if the pressure decreases at least 15%, we continue treatment. If the pressure does not decrease at least 15% we usually discontinue treatment and follow up on the patient's course without treatment. Medium-risk suspects are followed the same way as patients with early glaucoma (Table 5-1, page 100).

High-risk suspects with ocular hypertension. Although not everyone with high pressure has glaucoma, the greater the IOP for any given degree of nerve cupping, the greater the chance a person will demonstrate progressive disease. The assumption that the pressure at the time of diagnosis has been present for some time applies to glaucoma suspects as well as to individuals with manifest glaucoma; patients with highly elevated pressure without definite structural and functional damage usually have high thresholds for damage. However, the potential damage, if the assumption proves false, increases with increasing pressure. High-risk suspect patients have a CCT ≤ 555 microns, plus an IOP > 26 mmHg, cupping > 0.3, or both.

Try to lower the pressure in these high-risk individuals unless, after a discussion of their condition, they specifically oppose it. The goal of treatment is to decrease the risk of rapid damage and conversion to manifest glaucoma, not to achieve some normal pressure reading. Be careful not to pursue a course of expensive, annoying, or risky therapy for a clinical condition that is less threatening than mild, but fully manifest, glaucoma. As when treating other glaucoma suspects, we use medication only if it is well-tolerated. Our first choice is either a prostaglandin analog or a beta-blocker. High-risk suspects are followed the same way as patients with early glaucoma (Table 5-1, page 100).

Target Pressure in Glaucoma Suspect with Ocular Hypertension

We set the target pressure for a glaucoma suspect with ocular hypertension, if treatment is indicated, to a 15% reduction from baseline average.[*]

Chart 6-1 outlines the risk stratification and management approach for glaucoma suspect due to ocular hypertension.

---

[*] The Ocular Hypertension Treatment Study enrolled adults over the age of 40 years with enrollment IOP of 24-32 mmHg, and randomized patients to either observation or treatment. In the treatment group, a 20% reduction of average IOP with medication reduced the risk to glaucoma conversion by 36% in whites and 58% in blacks compared to the observation arm. [2,3]

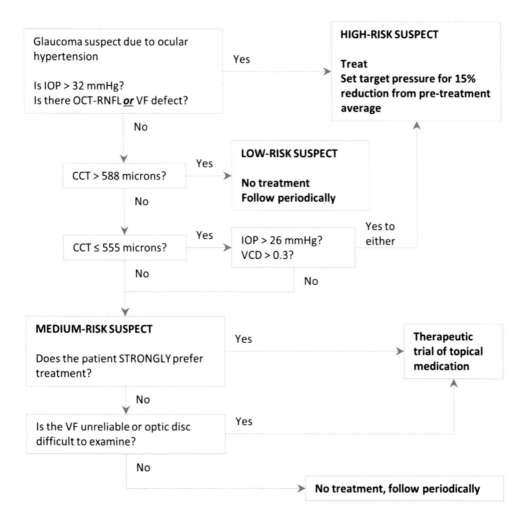

CHART 6-1. Steps in determining the risk of glaucoma conversion and the recommended management approach in a glaucoma suspect due to ocular hypertension. Key – OCT-RNFL (optical coherence tomography analysis of circumpapillary retinal nerve fiber layer), CCT (central corneal thickness), IOP (intraocular pressure), VCD (vertical cup/disc ratio), VF (visual field).

References

1. Gordon MO, Beiser JA, Brandt JD, et al. The Ocular Hypertension Study: baseline factors that predict the onset of primary open angle glaucoma. Archives of Ophthalmology. 2002; 120:714–720.

2. Palmberg P. How clinical trial results are changing our thinking about target pressures. Current Opinion in Ophthalmology. 2002 Apr;13(2):85-8.

3. Palmberg P. Evidence-based target pressures: how to choose and achieve them. International Ophthalmology Clinics. 2004 Spring;44(2):1-14.

7 GLAUCOMA SUSPECT II: ABNORMAL OPTIC DISC AND/OR VISUAL FIELD FINDINGS

All patients with glaucoma have optic nerve damage, but not all optic nerve damage is glaucomatous. The nerve fiber bundle defect is the hallmark of glaucoma, but not every nerve fiber bundle defect is caused by glaucoma. In the absence of significantly elevated pressure, the presence of optic nerve cupping or an unexplained visual field defect warrants a careful evaluation. The diagnostic possibilities of greatest immediate concern when a patient is first seen with an abnormal field or disc are treatable neurologic conditions, particularly tumors, and treatable vascular conditions such as cranial arteritis. Other fairly common conditions include nonarteritic vascular conditions, glaucoma with labile pressures, and past elevated pressure with resultant damage. These conditions must be recognized because their management differs from that of glaucoma.

A glaucoma suspect with low baseline IOP has cupping consistent with glaucoma, retinal nerve fiber layer (RNFL) loss, field loss, or some combination of these findings, with intraocular pressures (IOP) consistently less than 22 mmHg. As mentioned in Chapter 3, when the baseline IOP is low, we do not always presume the glaucomatous process to be present or active, although it very well may be. Previously categorized as "normal tension glaucoma," we do not believe glaucoma with low baseline IOP to be a distinct entity from high-pressure forms of open angle glaucoma, although this group of patients may require additional neuro-ophthalmologic workup.

In general, patients without elevated IOP are identified as glaucoma suspects in one of two ways. The clinician may note suspicious cupping during a routine examination of a person with normal IOP, or the patient may note a visual symptom and come to the doctor, who performs a field examination that shows a field defect. Occasionally, an asymptomatic person has a routine screening visual field test that shows a defect or has a RNFL abnormality noted on slit lamp exam and/or optical coherence tomography (OCT).

The following discussion concerns those patients in whom another diagnosis is not immediately obvious and in whom glaucoma is a possibility. We do not discuss patients in whom a routine evaluation leads to a clear diagnosis, for example those with bitemporal hemianopsia or acute and obvious retinal vascular occlusions. The evaluation of a glaucoma suspect with low baseline IOP proceeds as does the evaluation of a person with elevated IOP. The goal is to identify those individuals who have some recognizable condition and particularly to recognize those individuals who have treatable conditions. As mentioned previously (page 62), nonglaucomatous etiologies should be carefully considered if a glaucoma suspect with normal IOP has any of the following –

- Age < 50 years
- Best-corrected vision worse than 20/40 (and out of proportion to media clarity)

- Optic disc pallor greater than cupping
- Visual field with borderline vertical midline defect
- Non-migraine headaches and/or localizing neurologic symptoms

Evaluating the Patient

History: Asymptomatic Patient

Birth history. This may be difficult to obtain in most adult patients, unless the birth parents are present to provide the information. However, when available, a history of perinatal complications (e.g. intracranial hemorrhage, hydrocephalus, etc.) or prematurity may be associated with optic atrophy that presents as non-progressive cupping of the optic disc, though careful follow-up is required to demonstrate stability.

Systemic hypotension. Shock or marked systemic hypotension sometimes causes optic nerve damage and field loss that mimic glaucoma. Ask about injuries, previous blood transfusions, hypotensive episodes during surgery, hospitalization with intensive care, etc. Damage caused by hypotension rarely progresses. Because it is usually impossible to be certain, even in a person with a history of shock, that the ocular findings and medical history are related, these patients remain glaucoma suspects and require follow-up.

Possible previous pressure elevations. Prior use of topical or systemic corticosteroids or past surgery or injury may have temporarily caused elevated pressure. A patient who is using systemic beta-blockers may have had elevated IOP before using the medication. Pigment dispersion may have caused a pressure elevation in earlier years.

Vasospasm. Migraine is associated with glaucoma with low baseline IOP. Other vasospastic conditions such as Raynaud's phenomenon also appear to be associated with this type of glaucoma.

Family history. Primary open angle glaucoma with elevated and with low baseline IOP may mingle within the same family. Ask not only whether relatives have glaucoma, but also try to determine the severity of any disease uncovered. Alternatively, increased physiologic cupping may be familial[1] and a history of family members being monitored as "glaucoma suspects" without treatment may suggest that cupping is physiologic rather than pathologic.

History: Symptomatic Patient

In addition to checking the history-related points mentioned, question a patient with a symptomatic visual field defect about the onset (date, circumstances, associated symptoms) of the defect and about its subsequent course. A significant visual field defect that had a sudden onset is unlikely to be related to glaucoma, and the major immediate diagnostic concern in this setting is cranial arteritis for which the patient should be evaluated. A visual annoyance noted some time ago that has worsened may be glaucoma, but compressive lesions also progress.

Examination

Visual acuity. The best corrected visual acuity guides the evaluation of cupping and field loss. Until late in the disease, glaucoma rarely decreases the Snellen acuity significantly, whereas mass lesions involving the optic nerve often affect the acuity.

Color vision. Test color vision in each eye using standard pseudoisochromatic plates such as the Ishihara or Hardy-Rand-Rittler. Severely impaired color vision suggests inflammatory, compressive or infiltrative optic neuropathies, while it is rare finding in early or moderate glaucoma.[2,3]

Visual fields. Perform a central 24° static threshold field examination. If the acuity is unexpectedly reduced or if the patient complains of central visual symptoms, perform an Amsler grid examination before ocular manipulation. Examine the field carefully for atypical features, especially for central scotomas (look at the foveal threshold value) and for asymmetry across the vertical midline. Typical nerve fiber bundle defects that cross the vertical midline occur in patients with glaucoma, disc drusen, and anterior ischemic optic neuropathy. Central scotomas do not generally occur in glaucoma and suggest optic nerve compression; vertical hemianopic defects cannot be attributed to glaucoma. For a symptomatic patient with a normal 24° visual field, perform a 10° field.

Slit-lamp examination. Look for evidence of conditions that may have elevated the pressure in the past, such as trauma or previous inflammation. Also check for conditions that may be associated with intermittent pressure elevations, such as pigment dispersion, pseudoexfoliation, or narrow angles. Examine the lens carefully to rule out spherophakia and phacodonesis, which can cause intermittent pupillary block even when the angles are wide open at other times.

Tonometry. If some method other than applanation was used to check the pressure, repeat the measurement with an applanation tonometer. A number of pressure measurements on different days and different times of day may detect a variable, sometimes elevated pressure. Both for diagnosis and as part of a baseline examination, we suggest that measurements be done on at least 3 different days.

Gonioscopy. Examine the angle for evidence of previous events, such as trauma and inflammation, and for evidence of possible intermittent angle closure. Evaluate for and, if present, relieve any possible pupillary block as described in Chapter 2. A narrow angle can exist coincidentally with any other ocular or systemic abnormality, but significant pupillary block in this setting should be treated.

Ophthalmoscopy –

Disc examination. Examine the optic discs using a magnified binocular system and a slit beam as described in Chapter 2. There are no pathognomonic findings for a glaucomatous disc, although the following suggest acquired damage:

- Vertical cupping greater than 0.7 disc diameter.
- Asymmetry between the two cups of 0.2 disc diameters or greater in either axis in discs of equal size (Figure 7-1 A, B).
- Vertical elongation of the cup such that the vertical cup measurement is greater than the horizontal (Figure 7-1 C).
- A thinner rim in a vertical pole of the disc than elsewhere (Figure 7-1 D).
- Distinct local notching of the nerve tissue (Figure 7-1 E).
- Disc margin hemorrhage (Figure 7-1 F).

Pallor disproportionate to cupping, especially an area of focal pallor corresponding to a field defect, suggests a nonglaucomatous cause (Figure 7-2). Drusen of the nerve head may cause field defects, and if suspected but not seen may be confirmed with echography. Shunt vessels on the disc suggest a previous retinal vein obstruction (Figure 7-3). Anomalous or hypoplastic discs may be associated with visual field defects (Figure 7-4). Horizontal cupping greater than vertical cupping can be seen in some variants of optic nerve hypoplasia (Figure 7-5).

Retinal findings. Examine the retina carefully for retinal scars that could produce field defects, for subtle staphylomas, and for signs of previous vascular occlusion, such as vascular attenuation, shunt vessels, and peripheral hemorrhages.

Retinal Nerve Fiber Layer Imaging

The interpretation of OCT-RNFL analyses is discussed in Chapter 2. An optic disc with a large cup but normal RNFL thickness and contour is likely to be physiologic, and comparable thickness/contour in asymmetric cupping can rule out the large cup being pathologic (Figures 7-6, 7-7). However, the absence of progressive optic disc changes can only be ruled out with serial follow-up, even if the initial scan is normal.

A

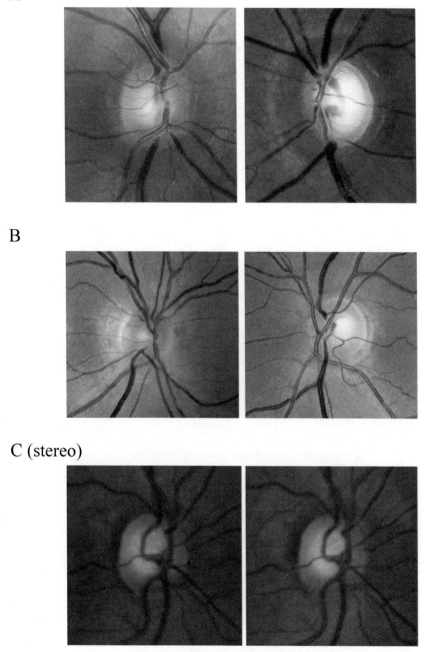

B

C (stereo)

FIG 7-1. Optic disc findings suggestive of glaucoma. **A.** Cup asymmetry in nerves of equal size. This patient has severe glaucoma in the left eye. **B.** Cup asymmetry in nerves of different size. The patient does not have glaucoma. **C.** Stereo photos showing vertical elongation of the cup (*continued next page*).

D (stereo)

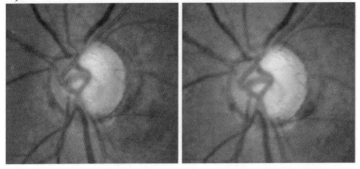

E (stereo)

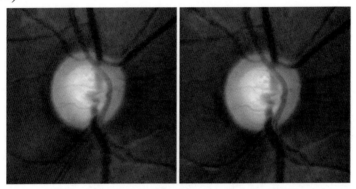

F

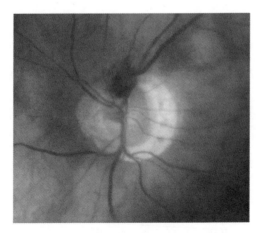

FIG 7-1. Optic disc findings suggestive of glaucoma (*continued*). **D.** Stereo photos showing thinning of the rim at the superior and inferior poles of the disc. **E.** Stereo photos showing inferior notching of the neuroretinal rim. **F.** Disc margin hemorrhage.

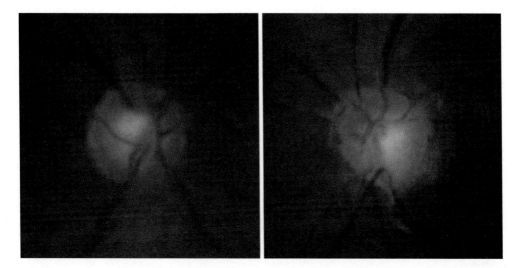

FIG 7-2. Pallor out of proportion to cupping. This patient had the sudden onset of a superior altitudinal defect in the left eye after cataract surgery and was diagnosed with nonarteritic anterior ischemic optic neuropathy. The photos show a normal right optic nerve with inferior pallor in the left optic nerve.

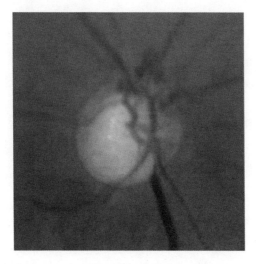

FIG 7-3. Shunt vessels in a patient with a field defect and a previous central retinal vein occlusion. This patient also has pre-existing glaucoma.

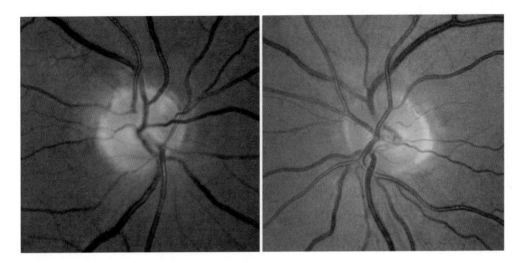

FIG 7-4. Hypoplastic discs in a patient with a field defect.

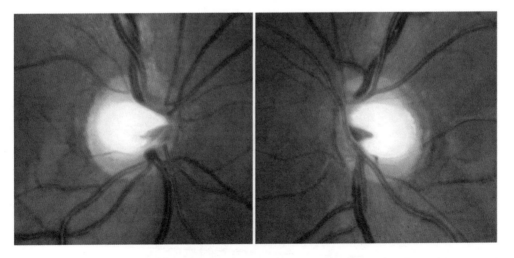

FIG 7-5. Horizontal cupping in optic nerve hypoplasia. This young patient has bitemporal hemianopsia and neuroimaging revealed chiasmal and optic nerve hypoplasia. The disc appearance, visual fields and retinal nerve fiber layer analyses have been stable for 3 years without treatment.

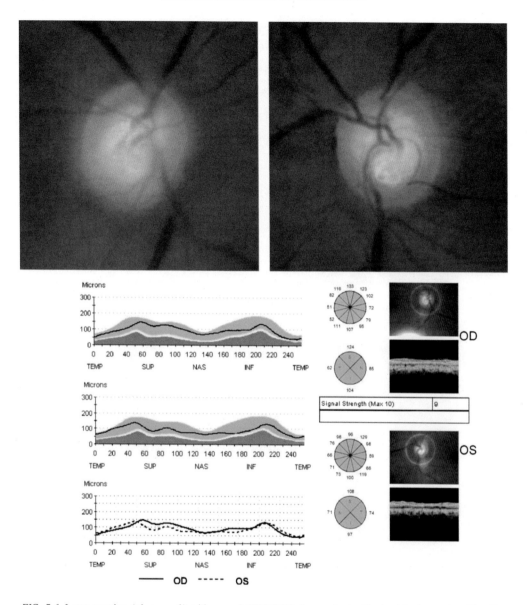

FIG. 7-6. Large cupping (*photograph*) with normal OCT-RNFL in a patient with physiologic cupping. The disc appearances and OCT-RNFL have remained unchanged without treatment over a 3-year follow-up.

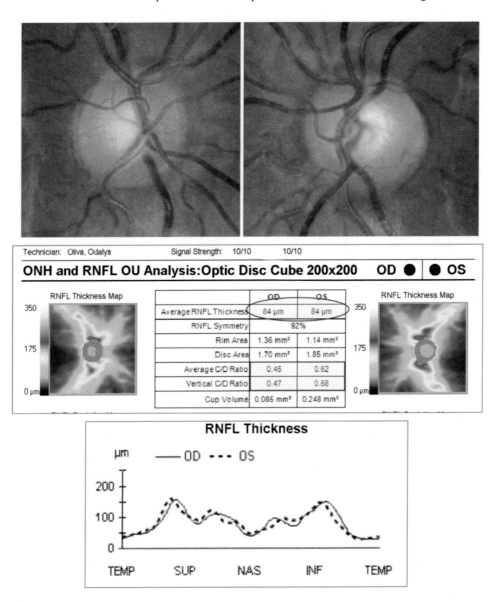

FIG. 7-7. Physiologically asymmetric cupping. The left eye has larger disc and cup compared to the fellow eye. While the average and vertical cup/disc ratios differ (*red rectangle*), the average circumpapillary retinal nerve fiber layer thicknesses are comparable with nearly identical contours (*red oval*).

Evaluating Possible Glaucomatous Cupping with Low Baseline IOP

Chart 7-1 summarizes the diagnostic steps in patients with low IOP suspected of having glaucoma.

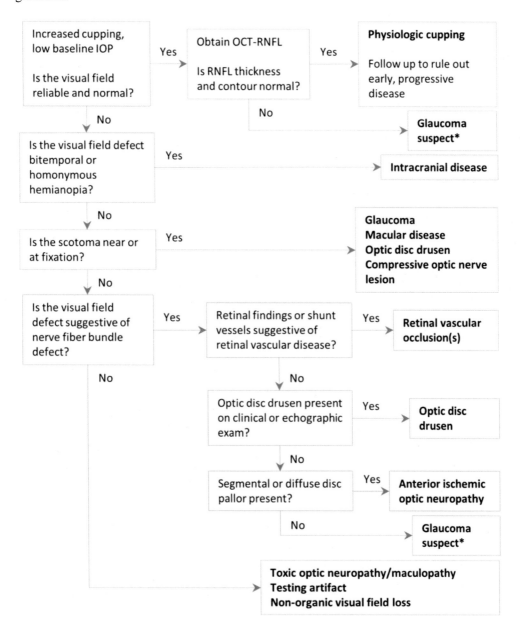

CHART 7-1. Differential diagnosis of glaucoma suspects with low baseline IOP. Key – OCT-RNFL (optical coherence tomographic analysis of retinal nerve fiber layer), IOP (intraocular pressure). *A glaucoma suspect is monitored more frequently than a patient with physiologic cupping to rule out progressive structural and/or functional changes and conversion to manifest glaucoma.

Differential Diagnoses

Cupping, normal visual field. If there are no other disc findings, such as hemorrhages, and if the neuroretinal rim is intact and of good color, the most likely diagnosis is large physiologic cupping. An OCT-RNFL with normal thickness and contour supports the diagnosis of physiologic cupping, although early glaucoma cannot be ruled out without serial scans demonstrating stability. Glaucoma without detected field loss is more likely if the disc has any of the other findings supporting glaucoma.

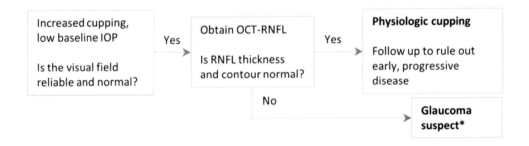

Cupping, visual field with bitemporal or homonymous hemianopia. These defects indicate disease at or behind the chiasm. Although pallor alone generally accompanies descending optic atrophy, cupping may also develop, or generous physiologic cupping may have been present beforehand.

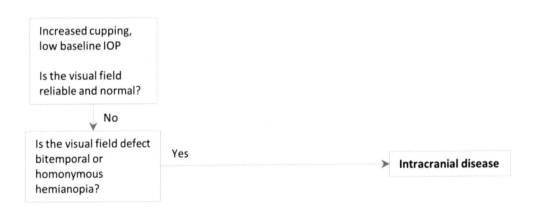

Cupping, visual field with scotoma at or near fixation. Although paracentral scotomas occur frequently in individuals who have glaucoma with low baseline IOP, central scotomas are not common. Central scotomas associated with cupping may be caused by compression of the optic nerve. Pallor of the nerve disproportionate to the cupping also suggests nerve compression in the presence of generous physiologic cupping. If neither the Amsler grid examination nor a careful macular examination reveals maculopathy to explain central field loss, it is appropriate to investigate the optic nerve with echography, neuroradiologic imaging, or both, particularly in unilateral cases. Myopic eyes (perhaps with a temporal crescent) may have scotomas affecting fixation early in the course of glaucoma.

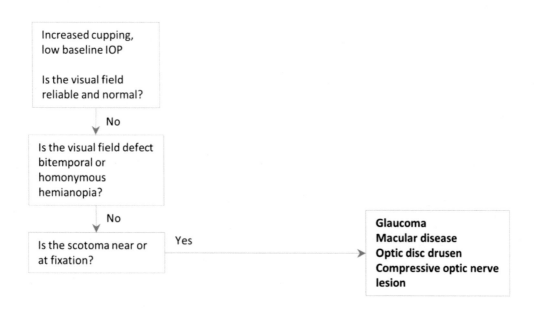

Cupping, visual field with defect suggesting nerve fiber bundle damage. Defects due to nerve fiber bundle damage crossing the vertical midline are always prechiasmal and usually indicate a lesion at the nerve head or in the retina. Retinal vascular causes, such as branch arterial occlusions and anterior ischemic optic neuropathy, are visible on fundus examination when acute, but after the early signs resolve they may be difficult to recognize. These conditions mimic glaucoma when they occur in patients with large physiologic cupping. Examine the vessels for thinning and the retinal pigment epithelium for local derangement. Segmental pallor of the nerve in the area corresponding to the field defect suggests a vascular accident, as does a history of acute field loss.

Field loss (with or without symptoms) without obvious cupping. The possible causes of field loss without abnormal cupping are the same as those with cupping, but glaucoma is much less likely than other conditions. Buried disc drusen may present in this fashion. Echography confirms or rules out the presence of drusen. In other cases, the nature of the field loss guides the diagnostic considerations.

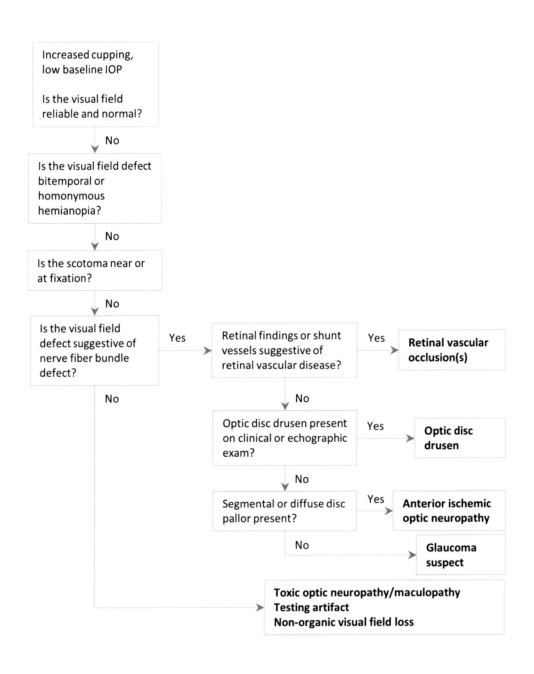

Symptoms suggesting scotoma without visual field loss. Routine perimetry may miss scotomas that fall between test points. Symptomatic scotomas are generally central or paracentral, and sometimes a patient can draw his or her scotoma on an Amsler grid chart. Depending on the character of the scotoma drawn, consider the above possibilities. If a 24-2 visual field test is unrevealing, perform a 10-2 visual field (Figure 7-8). If the patient has glaucoma, it will become apparent over time.

Neuroradiologic Investigation

In the setting of a glaucoma evaluation, we recommend appropriate neuroimaging for the following indications:

- Glaucomatous appearing cup with low baseline IOP and age < 50 years
- Unexplained decrease in visual acuity (central scotoma)
- Unusual visual field loss – field loss other than nerve fiber bundle defects
- Possibly bitemporal or homonymous hemianopic defects (clear defects also need evaluation, but they are not diagnostic dilemmas)
- Pallor disproportionate to cupping, unless the pallor is clearly confined to either the upper or lower half of the nerve (and thus likely related to a vascular event)
- Unilateral field loss not explained by obvious ocular asymmetry or concurrent unilateral disease

If a patient has normal Snellen acuity, glaucomatously cupped nerves, and bilateral nerve fiber bundle defects, we do not obtain imaging studies.

Medical Evaluation

General medical evaluation is usually unrewarding. It may reveal some treatable medical condition such as systemic hypertension or obstructive sleep apnea and perhaps patients are well served by finding a condition that deserves treatment in its own right. Only rarely is there a finding (such as a carotid occlusion of the side with worse visual loss) that seems related to the suspected glaucoma.

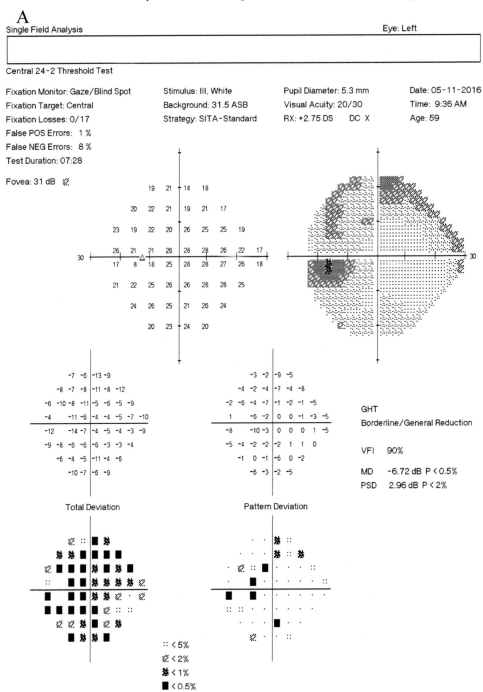

FIG 7-8. A 59 year-old woman being followed for glaucoma with normal IOP reports a new onset of symptoms suggestive of a central scotoma. **A.** (*this page*) the 24-2 field with generalized depression and nonspecific losses is stable from her prior studies and does not show a paracentral scotoma. Her visual acuity is 20/30, and foveal threshold is 31 dB. **B.** (*next page*) a 10-2 field performed later the same day shows a dense, central scotoma threatening fixation. Note that the 24-2 and 10-2 programs only overlap at one test point in each quadrant (Figure 2-15, page 32).

B

Single Field Analysis

Eye: Left

Central 10-2 Threshold Test

Fixation Monitor: Gaze/Blind Spot
Fixation Target: Central
Fixation Losses: 0/20
False POS Errors: 6 %
False NEG Errors: 0 %
Test Duration: 07:25

Fovea: 34 dB

Stimulus: III, White
Background: 31.5 ASB
Strategy: SITA-Standard

Pupil Diameter: 5.1 mm
Visual Acuity: 20/30
RX: +3.25 DS   DC X

Date: 05-11-2016
Time: 10:13 AM
Age: 59

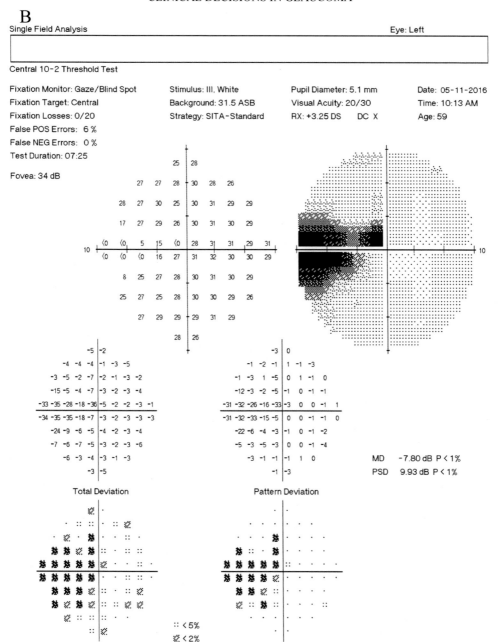

MD   -7.80 dB P < 1%
PSD   9.93 dB P < 1%

Total Deviation

Pattern Deviation

:: < 5%
⌧ < 2%
⬚ < 1%

Managing Glaucoma Suspects with Low Baseline IOP

Glaucoma suspects with low baseline IOP are managed much the same as glaucoma suspects with elevated IOP. The clinician should establish a baseline, determine the risk of progressive symptomatic glaucomatous damage, and decide whether to treat. If treatment is chosen, set a target pressure and attempt to achieve it. All patients should be observed for evidence of worsening.

Management Steps for Glaucoma Suspects

1. Establish a baseline.
2. Determine the risk of glaucomatous damage.
3. Decide whether to treat the IOP. If treatment is chosen, set a target pressure and attempt to achieve it.
4. Continue to observe all patients for evidence of worsening.

Baseline Examination

The baseline examination for glaucoma suspects with low baseline IOP is the same as for those with high baseline IOP and includes disc photos, OCT-RNFL analysis and a baseline set of threshold field examinations (Chapter 2). Obtain numerous pressure readings at different times in the day.

Determination of Risk

For purposes of determining risk and deciding whether to treat, there are two categories of individuals suspected of having glaucoma with low baseline IOP: those who have no field loss and those with abnormal fields. Risk in this context refers to the risk of having symptomatically significant damage develop without first having an asymptomatic defect develop that both alerts the clinician to the progressive nature of the condition and indicates the pace of damage. Risk does not mean something that can necessarily be changed by changing the pressure; the relative risks of untreated glaucoma occurring at low IOP versus the treatment necessary to lower pressure are not known.

Glaucoma suspects without field loss. All patients with normal IOP and normal visual fields are low-risk suspects. Even if field loss develops, it is unlikely to be symptomatic at its onset. Any change in such patients' conditions is likely to be slow.

Glaucoma suspects with field loss. Even if there are findings suggestive of progressive disease, such as a splinter hemorrhage, the risk to the patient relates to the pace of disease, which is not apparent at onset. When a glaucoma suspect has field loss, the location of the field loss guides the assessment of risk. The more severe the field loss, and particularly the closer a scotoma is to fixation, the greater the risk that detectable worsening from baseline will be visually critical; thus we are more aggressive in such cases.

We stratify glaucoma suspects with low baseline IOP as follows –

- Low-risk suspects – anyone with no or only early visual field loss <u>and</u> normal sensitivity within the central 5°.
- High-risk suspects – everyone else (either moderate or severe visual field loss, or anyone with abnormal sensitivity within the central 5°).

Establishing a Plan: Target Pressure and Treatment

The rationale outlined below is based on the findings of Collaborative Normal Tension Glaucoma Study (Chapter 4, page 77, footnote). Note that in order to achieve a treated IOP that is 30% lower than the pre-treatment baseline, we set a target pressure (the upper limit of the treated IOP range) that is 20% lower than the mean pre-treatment IOP.

Low-risk suspects. Follow these patients without therapy using the schedule for early glaucomatous defect in Chapter 5 (Table 5-1, page 100).

High-risk suspects. Regardless of whether high-risk suspects have pressure-related damage, they certainly have vision-threatening disease. After ruling out other treatable conditions, treat these patients with topical, laser, and/or oral therapy as needed to achieve at least a 20% reduction from mean pre-treatment IOP. If the pressure does not decrease at least 20%, the management plan is based on the extent of visual field loss. Those with moderate loss not threatening fixation can be monitored on maximum conservative therapy, while those with severe loss and/or threatened fixation may require incisional surgery. If fixation is threatened in both eyes, we do not do incisional surgery in both eyes until it is apparent that the eye with surgery has fared better. Follow these patients using the schedule for patients with moderate or severe glaucomatous defect in Chapter 5 (Table 5-1, page 100)

If a glaucoma suspect with low baseline IOP, either treated or untreated, demonstrates progressive damage, evaluate the patient to ensure that the progression does not suggest some nonglaucomatous process. If no other explanation is found and the findings are consistent with glaucoma, then the patient has manifest glaucoma. The follow-up of manifest glaucoma is discussed in Chapter 5.

Reference

1. Chang TC, Congdon NG, Wojciechowski R, Muñoz B, Gilbert D, Chen P, Friedman DS, West SK. Determinants and heritability of intraocular pressure and cup-to-disc ratio in a defined older population. Ophthalmology. 2005 Jul;112(7):1186-91.

2. Hamill TR, Post RB, Johnson CA, Keltner JL. Correlation of color vision deficits and observable changes in the optic disc in a population of ocular hypertensives. Archi ves of ophthalmology. 1984 Nov;102(11):1637-9.

3. Miller NR, Newman NJ, eds. *Walsh & Hoyt's Clinical Neuro-Ophthalmology, 5th Edition: The Essentials*. Baltimore: Williams & Wilkins, 1999. Print.

8 GLAUCOMA SUSPECT III: THE ABNORMAL ANGLE

This chapter discusses patients who have not had surgery in whom the gonioscopic findings alone suggest that glaucoma may develop. Although there are many possible abnormal gonioscopic findings, the common conditions that fit this category include: narrow angle, dense pigmentation of the trabecular meshwork, congenital anomalies such as the Axenfeld-Rieger syndrome, and angle recession.

Narrow Angle

The nomenclature of the narrow angle has evolved since the first edition of this book.[1] We categorize patients with narrow angles into the following categories –

- Primary angle closure glaucoma – manifest glaucoma which occurs in an eye with less than 180° of visible trabecular meshwork on gonioscopy.
- Primary angle closure – intraocular pressure (IOP) > 21 mmHg and/or peripheral anterior synechiae (PAS) in an eye with less than 180° of visible trabecular meshwork on gonioscopy, with normal visual fields, optic discs and retinal nerve fiber layer analysis on optical coherence tomography.
- Primary angle closure suspect – a person with at least one eye with less than 180 degrees of visible trabecular meshwork on gonioscopy, no glaucoma, no PAS, and normal IOP.

Most primary angle closure suspects do not develop either acute or chronic angle closure glaucoma. However, such glaucoma almost always occurs in eyes with primary angle closure.[*] None of the various provocative tests introduced over the years accurately predicts who will have spontaneous closure.

Evaluate and rule out secondary causes of a narrow angle, such as ciliary body swelling (related to sulfonamide use, central retinal or vortex vein occlusion, uveal effusion syndrome), lens abnormalities (loose zonules, spherophakia, lens intumescence), iridocorneal endothelial dystrophy, and intraocular tumors.

An iridotomy can alleviate and/or prevent angle closure due to pupillary block. It does not necessarily prevent angle closure from other causes, and chronic angle closure glaucoma due to other mechanisms can still occur in the setting of a patent iridotomy.

We perform iridotomy on asymptomatic primary angle closure suspects who fit any of the following categories:

---

[*] In a prospective, observational study, approximately 20% of untreated primary angle closure suspects developed either ocular hypertension and/or peripheral anterior synechiae over 5 years, though none developed any glaucomatous damage. [1]

- Progression to primary angle closure, with or without glaucoma
- Elevated IOP and angle closure that develops when the pupils are dilated[**]
- Acute or chronic angle closure in the other eye
- Transient symptoms typical for self-limited attacks of angle closure
- Inability to be evaluated promptly if symptoms develop
- Posterior pole comorbidities, such as diabetic retinopathy, that require frequent dilated fundus examinations
- Significant patient anxiety about the risk of spontaneous acute angle closure

Dense Pigmentation of the Trabecular Meshwork

Pigment dispersion and pseudoexfoliation are the most common causes of increased pigmentation. As noted in Chapter 2, unilateral pigmentation is sometimes caused by a lens implant that chafes against the iris and is very rarely caused by a tumor that sheds cells into the eye. In the absence of other indications of glaucoma, neither pigmentary dispersion nor the pseudoexfoliation syndrome without elevated pressure demands special treatment.

Congenital Anomalies such as Axenfeld-Rieger Syndrome

Individuals with congenital anomalies of the anterior segment who do not have glaucoma or elevated pressure should have an ophthalmic examination at least yearly.

Angle Recession

A patient who is noted to have an angle recession on routine examination has a higher chance of developing glaucoma than a similar person without a recession. The likelihood depends on the degree of the initial trauma to the anterior segment as well as on the patient's underlying outflow dynamics. There is no precise amount of angle recession that decrees glaucoma in the future nor is there a degree of recession below which the practitioner need not worry.[*] A history of trauma, not the finding of angle recession, confers increased risk of secondary glaucoma. Hence, a known history of blunt trauma is enough to require life-long follow-up even if angle recession is absent.

Always examine the rest of the eye for other evidence of trauma. We recommend a diagnostic visual field examination to identify possible visual field effects related to the injury. Obtain baseline optic disc imaging studies, and reexamine the patient yearly.

[**] The purpose of the iridotomy is to allow for prompt and safe dilation if the patient develops an ocular complaint, not because closure after pharmacologic dilation predicts spontaneous angle closure.

[*] In a population-based glaucoma survey, angle recession was noted unilaterally in 6% and bilaterally in 9% of screened participants. Prevalence of glaucoma was 5.5% in eyes with any angle recession, and 8% in eyes with 360° of angle recession. [2]

References

1. Thomas R, George R, Parikh R, Muliyil J, Jacob A. Five year risk of progression of primary angle closure suspects to primary angle closure: a population based study. British Journal of Ophthalmology. 2003 Apr;87(4):450-4.

2. Salmon JF, Mermoud A, Ivey A, Swanevelder SA, Hoffman M. The detection of post-traumatic angle recession by gonioscopy in a population-based glaucoma survey. Ophthalmology. 1994 Nov;101(11):1844-50.

9 ACUTE SYMPTOMATIC ELEVATED INTRAOCULAR PRESSURE

The patient who is initially seen with a sudden onset of symptoms (other than field loss) caused by high intraocular pressure (IOP) may have any type of pathology that produces markedly elevated pressure. Corneal edema, which causes blurring and halos, and ciliary spasm, which causes deep, aching pain, may result from either an acute process that produces a sudden, severe pressure increase or from a chronic pressure elevation that eventually becomes high enough to produce anterior segment ischemia.

Although the *possible* diagnoses include almost all types of glaucoma, there are only a few likely diagnostic possibilities. The most common are:

- Acute angle closure (due to pupillary block or other etiology)
- Chronic angle closure with acute decompensation
- Neovascularization of the angle
- Pseudoexfoliation syndrome
- Pigment dispersion syndrome
- Ocular hypertension resulting from old trauma
- Glaucomatocyclitic crisis

Acute, symptomatically elevated IOP frequently, but not always, leads to glaucomatous damage of the optic nerve. We use the term "glaucoma" when glaucomatous optic nerve damage is suspected or demonstrated. Otherwise, we describe the condition based on the identifiable pathophysiology. Patients with these conditions usually have acute symptoms in only one eye, and the history and physical examination usually allow accurate diagnosis and identification of those patients who do not "fit" one of the usual categories.

Making a Diagnosis

History

Although the diagnosis depends on the physical examination in this group of patients, the history and circumstances of presentation provide clues that may suggest a specific cause of high pressure. None of these clues is absolute, but they are helpful. The typical presentation for each of the likely conditions follows. For patients with acute, symptomatic elevated IOP following surgery (either early or late in the postoperative course), see Chapter 11.

Acute and chronic angle closure. This condition is more common in women than men. Most patients are older than 60 years of age. Almost all patients with acute angle closure are hyperopic. Some have histories of transient episodes of pain or blurred vision in one or both eyes. If these symptoms occurred in relation to pupillary dilation, such as while sitting in a darkened theater, and resolved with pupillary constriction, such as upon entering the lobby, the diagnosis is very likely. Patients with chronic angle closure do not have histories of such episodes. Rarely, acute angle closure secondary to ciliary body edema and anterior rotation of the lens-iris diaphragm may be precipitated by certain sulfa-based systemic medications, such as topiramate or acetazolamide. [1]

Neovascularization of the angle. Most previously undiagnosed people who have neovascularization of the angle have either proliferative diabetic retinopathy or have had a central retinal vein occlusion. Those with diabetic retinopathy usually know that they have diabetes, but may be unaware of any eye disease. Individuals with juvenile onset diabetes usually have had their disease more than 10 years. Those with central retinal vein occlusions usually have noticed a decrease in their vision within the previous 2 to 4 months. Many of these patients have hypertension.

Pseudoexfoliation syndrome. These patients are rarely younger than 65 years of age. The elevated IOP may be due to either a secondary open angle mechanism, presumably from accumulation of the pseudoexfoliation material in the angle, or a lenticular-pupillary block mechanism with secondary angle closure from zonular laxity and anterior movement of the lens.

Pigment dispersion syndrome. This condition generally occurs in moderately myopic men who are younger than 50. They often describe transient episodes of blurred vision or of seeing halos around lights, particularly after exercise. These episodes are probably caused by elevated pressure related to a shower of pigment in the anterior chamber.

Old trauma. Trauma is more common in men than in women. The injury may have occurred decades before presentation and may be forgotten.

Glaucomatocyclitic crisis. Patients with this condition may be of any age, but most patients are seen before the age of 60. There is no refractive or gender predilection. Patients may have a history of previous episodes of painless blurring without ocular injection, sometimes in the eye not involved in the episode that prompts medical attention.

Examination

The physical examination allows accurate diagnosis of most cases of acute pressure elevation. The salient points of the various aspects of the examination are as follows:

Vision. Corneal edema may decrease the acuity markedly. If the acuity is good, central retinal vein occlusion with neovascular glaucoma is highly unlikely.

Pupils. When the pressure is high, the pupil often is mid-dilated and nonreactive or sluggish because of iris ischemia. The presence or absence of an afferent defect does not provide useful differential diagnostic information.

Slit lamp examination. If corneal edema obscures the view, topical glycerin may allow adequate biomicroscopy and gonioscopy.

Cornea. The presence of a Krukenberg spindle suggests pigmentary glaucoma. Diffuse pigment dusting (heavy or scant) can be found in both pigment dispersion and pseudoexfoliation.

Anterior chamber. Note the depth of the central anterior chamber and compare it with the opposite eye. If the lens has moved forward and caused angle closure while the opposite eye has a deeper chamber and a seemingly nonoccludable angle, consider pseudoexfoliation, traumatic subluxation of the lens, or ciliary body forward rotation. To supplement gonioscopy, it is often helpful to examine the peripheral anterior chamber with a narrow, well-focused slit beam. Even when the cornea is edematous, it may be possible to detect that the peripheral iris is in tight contact with the peripheral corneal endothelium, confirming angle closure. If the peripheral iris is distant from the cornea, this finding suggests secondary open angle pressure elevation.

If there is mild inflammation in conjunction with a normal iris and an open angle in this setting, the most likely diagnosis is glaucomatocyclitic crisis. The evidence of inflammation in glaucomatocyclitic crisis may be minimal initially, with only a mild flare and a few cells on presentation. The typical keratic precipitates may not appear until several days into the course. If there is substantial anterior segment inflammation, refer to Chapter 10.

Iris. Neovascularization is usually visible around the pupillary border if anterior segment neovascularization is the cause of acutely elevated pressure. If there is evidence of trauma (sphincter rupture is probably the most common finding) associated with an open angle, then acute pressure elevation related to angle contusion is the likely diagnosis. Inspect the iris carefully for transillumination defects either near the pupillary margin (pseudoexfoliation) or in the mid-periphery (pigment dispersion). Occasionally, pseudoexfoliation syndrome may present with minimal exfoliative deposits along the iris border that are easily missed.

Lens. Phacodonesis suggests either old trauma or, occasionally, pseudoexfoliation. Exfoliative material may be visible on the lens surface.

Gonioscopy. Many patients will have corneal edema, which renders gonioscopy difficult. If application of topical glycerin does not clear the view, it is often useful to perform gonioscopy on the uninvolved eye, as the angle configuration is often similar between the two eyes. If the angle is closed, perform indentation gonioscopy, which not only helps confirm that the angle is closed by revealing the structures in the artificially opened angle, but may reveal peripheral anterior synechiae (PAS), which indicate a chronic process causing the acute symptoms.

Funduscopy. Fundus evaluation, particularly if it precedes dilation, is often difficult in a photophobic patient who has corneal edema. If it is possible to see the fundus, note if the disc is swollen from an acute pressure rise or is cupped from a chronic pressure elevation with acute symptoms related to anterior segment decompensation. Try to determine the retinal causes of rubeosis iridis in cases of anterior segment neovascularization.

Differential Diagnosis

Chart 9-1 outlines the steps in gonioscopic diagnosis of the conditions that commonly present with symptomatic pressure elevations.

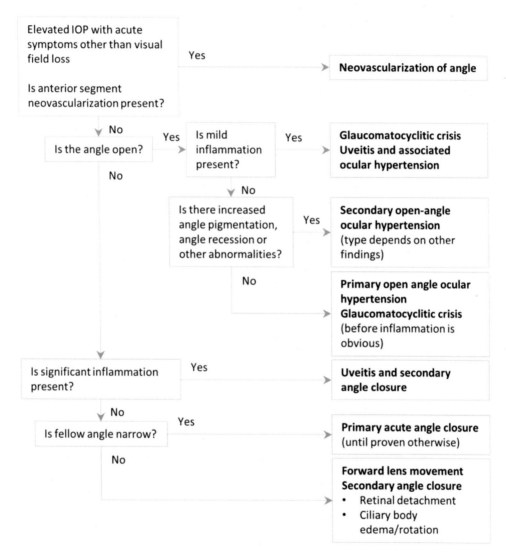

CHART 9-1. Differential diagnosis of the common causes of acute symptomatic elevated pressure. Key – IOP (intraocular pressure).

Angle neovascularization. If the angle is either closed with neovascularization or is open but contains a neovascular network over the trabecular meshwork, evaluate the posterior segment (funduscopy, echography) to clarify the cause of the neovascularization.

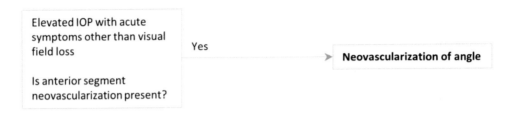

No neovascularization, angle open. Mild anterior segment inflammation suggests glaucomatocyclitic crisis and at times the inflammation is not apparent initially. Other uveitides may present acutely and are discussed in Chapter 10.

If the angle is open without neovascularization and the anterior chamber is quiet, look carefully for pigmentation and for evidence of trauma. A densely pigmented trabecular meshwork is always found in pigmentary glaucoma and is often seen to a slightly less striking degree in pseudoexfoliation. Examine the eye carefully for evidence of trauma; compare the two eyes for help in distinguishing asymmetry in angle depth and pigmentation.

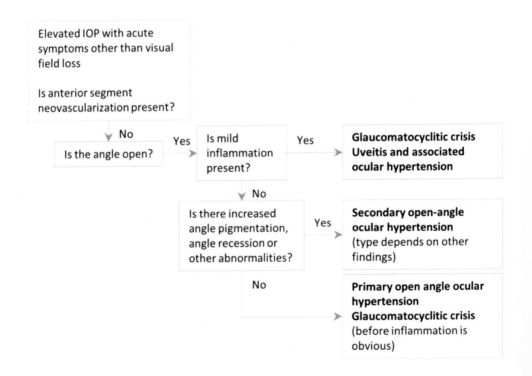

No neovascularization, angle closed. Angle closure in an eye with significant anterior segment inflammation is discussed in Chapter 10. Angle closure in an eye without significant anterior chamber reaction usually indicates primary acute angle closure. Unless the patient has, for example, anisometropia, the other eye usually has a very narrow angle. If the opposite eye has a narrow angle and peripheral anterior synechiae, then chronic angle closure with acute decompensation is likely. If the opposite angle is not narrow, then seek another explanation since other types of angle closure *may* present in this setting. If the central anterior chamber depth in the involved eye is distinctly shallower than in the other eye, the patient probably has a component of forward lens movement. This occurs in pseudoexfoliation, following trauma with lens subluxation, and occasionally as a drug reaction or as an isolated finding. In practice, forward lens movement, even if suspected, is usually confirmed after peripheral iridotomy.

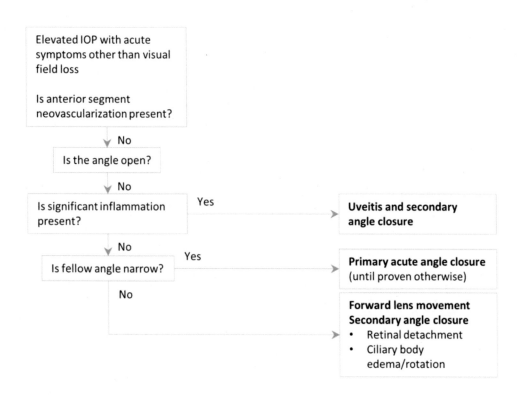

Treatment

Neovascularization of the Angle

Determination of mechanism. Proliferative diabetic retinopathy and recent central retinal vein occlusion are straightforward diagnoses in most cases. If neither of these possibilities seems reasonable, and if the physical examination reveals no cause, such as a choroidal tumor or a chronic retinal detachment, it is likely that there is no clear explanation. Neovascularization can occur secondary to chronic marked pressure elevation, as with untreated angle closure; it is important to examine the opposite eye for diagnostic clues. If none of the likely explanations appears to be accurate, the ocular ischemic syndrome is a default diagnosis in people with systemic vascular disease, in which case a neurovascular consultation is appropriate.

Treatment of underlying causes. Retinal ablation by photocoagulation is the definitive treatment of choice for both proliferative diabetic retinopathy and neovascularization related to central vein occlusions. Intraocular injection of anti-vascular endothelial growth factor (anti-VEGF) agents provides a fast-acting temporizing measure if the media is not sufficiently clear to permit thorough photocoagulation. If glaucoma surgery is planned, the treatment of neovascular etiologies ideally precedes glaucoma surgery, as active anterior segment neovascularization increases the risk of hyphema. However, if secondary angle-closure has already occurred and the IOP is markedly elevated despite medical therapy, we recommend prompt glaucoma surgery with concurrent intraoperative anti-VEGF therapy and/or retinal ablation. Medical therapy before ablation and while awaiting regression of the neovascularization includes anti-inflammatory agents and suppressants of aqueous humor formation. The following is a typical regimen:

- Topical atropine 1% twice daily
- Topical prednisolone acetate 1% four times daily
- Topical beta-blocker, alpha-agonist and/or carbonic anhydrase inhibitors twice daily
- (When necessary) systemic carbonic anhydrase inhibitor two to four times daily

After retinal ablation and/or intraocular anti-VEGF therapy, the degree of inflammation determines the duration of treatment with cycloplegic and corticosteroid drops. Management of the IOP is discussed in the next section.

If the neovascularization does not have an apparent explanation, we usually treat the patient medically for a few days to attempt to lower the pressure slightly and quiet the eye. We promptly seek consultation with a retina specialist. If there is substantial retinal nonperfusion, our retina consultants usually recommend retinal ablation. If the cause of neovascularization is presumed to be ocular ischemia related to systemic vascular (e.g. carotid) disease, then there is no well-established treatment, although such individuals often do have retinal ablation. The role of chronic intravitreal anti-VEGF therapy in the ocular ischemic syndrome is unknown.

Treatment of the IOP. Once the treatable causes of neovascularization have been managed, the residual eye pressure must be treated. The management depends on the response of the eye to ablation (if done) as well as to the pressure.

Regressed neovascularization. If the neovascularization regresses and the pressure falls to below 30 mmHg, treat the patient as a glaucoma suspect due to ocular hypertension as outlined in Chapter 6. If the pressure remains above 30 mmHg or if the optic nerve appears to be glaucomatously cupped, treat the patient as if he or she has manifest glaucoma; however, avoid miotics and do not perform laser trabeculoplasty. If surgery is indicated, implant a glaucoma drainage device (GDD). If repeated intraocular anti-VEGF injections are likely, we have a low threshold to implant a GDD as successful surgery blunts the expected episodic pressure elevations secondary to injections.

Persistent neovascularization. Active neovascularization suggests inadequate retinal ablation. Manage such patients according to the guidelines for the chronic care of uveitis with elevated pressure described in Chapter 10. If vitreoretinal surgery is warranted for endolaser ablation or other cause and the pressure is either borderline or above the desired target, we implant a GDD at the time of the vitreoretinal procedures.

Primary or Secondary Angle Closure

The management of acute angle closure involves immediate, early, and chronic steps.

Immediate treatment. The first treatment step is to lower the severely elevated IOP. Pressure reduction restores perfusion to the iris sphincter so it can respond to miotic drops. Three ways to lower the IOP are the administration of hyperosmotic agents, corneal indentation to force the angle open and allow aqueous humor to egress and, if there is sufficient room between the peripheral iris and the corneal endothelium, performance of a paracentesis. Two to three instillations of pilocarpine over 30 minutes will constrict the pupil if the pressure has been lowered. We treat patients with corticosteroid drops to quiet the eye, relieve symptoms, reduce synechiae formation, and prepare the eye for iridotomy.

During an acute episode of angle closure, the aqueous inflow almost ceases and suppressants of aqueous humor formation alone do not affect the pressure. After the pressure decreases and aqueous humor production resumes, such agents may be unnecessary if the angle is open and functional. However, it is reasonable to treat patients with a pressure-lowering medication until the functional status of the outflow system is known.

If a patient has acute angle closure and forward lens movement is suspected, treat the patient to lower the IOP but do not give miotic drops. Cycloplegic agents are appropriate treatment for forward lens movement, but it is preferable to perform an iridotomy to remove any possible pupillary block contribution before such drugs are used.

Early Treatment –

Relieve pupillary block. Perform a peripheral iridotomy in both the involved eye and, if it has a narrow angle, in the opposite eye. If the cornea is not clear enough for an iridotomy, maintain the patient on pilocarpine and examine him or her frequently while waiting for the cornea to clear sufficiently to allow laser treatment.

Gonioscopy. After performing the iridotomy, study the angle for clues to the patient's future course. PAS may have formed over an extended period of chronic angle closure or may have formed during a prolonged acute congestive attack. Synechiae directly block the egress of aqueous humor and raise the outflow pressure by about the same percentage as the angle is closed (see Chapter 4 for a discussion of outflow pressure). If forward lens movement caused the angle closure, the gonioscopic appearance after iridotomy does not change.

Dilate the pupil and examine the angle. If peripheral iridotomy does not relieve the angle closure and if forward lens movement is suspected, administer a cycloplegic agent, such as cyclopentolate 1%, and reexamine the eye. If the angle opens, the diagnosis of forward lens movement is confirmed. If cycloplegia does not relieve angle closure, plateau iris syndrome must be ruled out. This is an uncommon condition in which the angle remains closed or closes with dilation, despite the presence of a patent iridotomy. It is often difficult to diagnose this condition without checking the angle before and after dilation (although the appearance of ciliary processes on ultrasound biomicroscopy lends a clue, Figure 9-1). Treatment of a patient with plateau iris syndrome includes long-term miotic therapy and peripheral iris retraction (laser iridoplasty), which is described in standard surgical texts.

Examine the fundus. After angle closure has been treated, all patients should have a complete fundus examination if one has not already been performed.

A

B

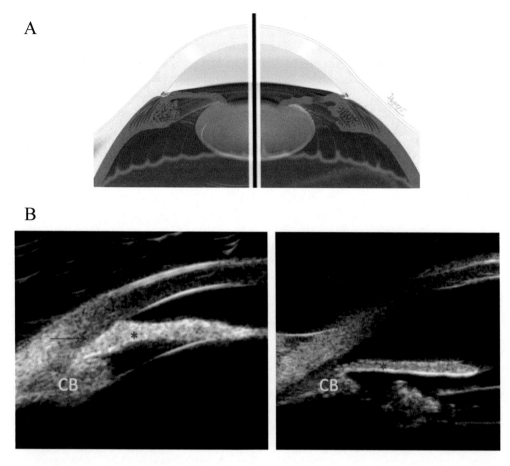

FIG 9-1. Plateau iris and angle closure. **A.** Proposed anatomic basis. The ciliary processes are more anterior than usual, and the peripheral iris drapes over them. Iridotomy does not alter the configuration because ciliary processes continue to support the iris, *left*. Normal anatomy for comparison, *right*. **B.** High-resolution anterior segment ultrasound appearance of plateau iris angle closure (*left*) and normal angle configuration for comparison (*right*). CB – ciliary body, asterisk – iris, arrow – closed angle.

Chronic treatment. After an attack of acute angle closure, the production of aqueous humor may be unusually low. This may be related to inflammation, but it resolves. Particularly if there are extensive PAS, it is important to observe the patient's condition carefully to determine whether the IOP rises as the formation of aqueous humor resumes. Appropriate follow-up depends on the IOP and the extent of PAS formation.

Normal pressure after early treatment. Peripheral anterior synechiae increase resistance to aqueous humor outflow and probably increase a patient's chance of developing elevated pressure with time. Even eyes with no synechiae may have damaged outflow systems. Thus we consider such patients to have a high risk of developing elevated pressure and examine them frequently early after the attack of angle closure. Disc imaging and visual fields should be performed on all patients once any disc swelling resolves to document the effects of the acute episode. We suggest the following graded management based on the extent of PAS:

- Low risk: less than 25% PAS. Examine the patient 6 and 18 months after the acute attack. If the pressure remains low and the eye appears stable, examine the patient every 1 to 2 years thereafter; further visual field examinations and imaging studies are not necessary.
- Medium risk: between 25 and 75% PAS. Examine the patient 4, 8, 12, and 24 months after the attack. If the pressure remains low and the eye appears stable, examine the patient every 1 to 2 years thereafter. The patient does not need to repeat the visual field examination or imaging studies.
- High risk: greater than 75% PAS. Examine the patient 3, 6, 9, 12, and 24 months after the attack. If the pressure remains low and the eye appears stable, examine the patient every year thereafter. Visual fields and imaging studies need not be repeated.

Elevated pressure after early treatment. If the pressure is elevated after iridotomy, determine the extent of PAS. Extensive synechiae may be treated with incisional synechialysis. Establish a baseline and begin chronic follow-up after such treatment.

One of the assumptions involved in managing individuals with asymptomatic elevated IOP – that they have had the same pressure as they have at diagnosis for some time – is clearly false in individuals after an acute angle closure attack. The pressure has not been elevated for an extended time. Most have had very high pressure for a short period and now have a lower, but still elevated, pressure. They may have manifest glaucoma, but their IOP without treatment, although still elevated, may now be safe for them.

Uncertainty regarding a patient's sensitivity to pressure dictates that the patient should have frequent examinations in the early years of follow-up. We suggest that the follow-up guides in Table 5-1 (page 100) be used with the adaptation that *everyone* be considered as having a severe glaucomatous defect for the first year. If the patient's condition remains stable, manage these patients as low or moderate risk suspects with elevated IOP by the recommended schedules (page 129).

Acute Secondary Open Angle Pressure Elevation

Pressure elevation due to either pseudoexfoliation or pigment dispersion is generally treated the same as primary open angle pressure elevation. However, when the presentation is that of an acute symptomatic pressure elevation, there are a few differences in the evaluation and management.

- It is not necessary to obtain several different pressure readings before starting treatment, because the IOP may be highly labile and the symptoms demand attention.
- It is reasonable to postpone obtaining a full baseline until the acute episode is resolved.

Even if the pressure is very high, avoid beginning more than one medication at a time. A person with corneal edema and pressures of 50 mmHg and 55 mmHg likely needs to have a lower pressure in each eye, but the patient does not need to achieve a pressure of 15 mmHg immediately. The higher the initial pressure, the greater will be the expected drop in pressure from the first medication. We usually administer a beta-blocker and have the patient stay in the office until the pressure starts to decrease. Within a day or so we re-examine the patient and consider whether to add more treatment. We obtain baseline fields and optic disc imaging after the acute episode passes and any nerve swelling has resolved.

Many patients with pseudoexfoliation or pigment dispersion who are seen initially with acute symptomatic glaucoma require laser or incisional surgery in the reasonably short term. However, we generally use the medication steps because some patients respond quite well. The chronic care of individuals with these conditions follows the guides in Chapters 4 and 5 with a few modifications discussed in Chapter 12.

Old Trauma

The medical management of acute open angle pressure elevation associated with old trauma is almost the same as that of primary open angle pressure elevation. Patients with a sufficiently elevated pressure to have acute symptoms often require surgery, but we treat them medically initially. Such patients do not need multiple IOP readings and visual fields before treatment. The clinician should treat to lower the pressure, usually with topical agents (miotics may work poorly) and then establish a baseline, etc. Treatment is much like that of patients with primary open angle pressure elevation with differences discussed in Chapter 12. If the IOP does not respond to initial topical medical treatments, we proceed with systemic carbonic anhydrase inhibitors and/or incisional surgery since laser treatment is rarely beneficial.

Glaucomatocyclitic Crisis

Treatment for glaucomatocyclitic crisis is discussed in Chapter 10.

Reference

1. Lachkar Y, Bouassida W. Drug-induced acute angle closure glaucoma. Current Opinion in Ophthalmology. 2007 Mar;18(2):129-33. Review.

10 UVEITIS AND ELEVATED PRESSURE

Uveitis encompasses a large, diverse group of conditions, many of which are accompanied by elevated intraocular pressure (IOP) at some point in their clinical course. In a particular patient with uveitis, the IOP may range from quite low to very high, because inflammation decreases both the rate of aqueous humor formation and the ease of aqueous humor exit from the eye. The balance between these two effects determines the pressure at any given time. The major causes of impaired outflow and thus elevated pressure are as follows:

- Temporary blockage of trabecular meshwork by inflammatory debris
- Peripheral anterior synechiae (PAS) formation related to organization of debris in the angle and gradual incorporation of the iris
- Appositional and then synechial angle closure caused by pupillary block from posterior synechiae formation
- Steroid-induced pressure elevation related to the treatment of ocular inflammation

The differential diagnosis, particular clinical features, and specific management of the various uveitides are beyond the scope of this book. Most patients with nontraumatic uveitis and elevated pressure have either idiopathic inflammation or a recognized syndrome that is managed in largely the same manner as idiopathic uveitis. Those with traumatic uveitis, following either surgical or nonsurgical trauma, are discussed in Chapter 11 and are managed similarly. However, management of the following syndromes is distinct from that of idiopathic uveitis:

- Glaucomatocyclitic crisis
- Fuchs heterochromic iridocyclitis
- Herpes zoster or simplex-associated uveitis
- Phacolytic and/or phacoantigenic glaucoma
- Ciliary body inflammation and rotation with angle closure glaucoma

One of the goals of the evaluation of patients with uveitis and elevated pressure is to recognize these conditions. A second goal is to recognize those patients who have one of the chronic uveitis syndromes, most commonly sarcoidosis or juvenile idiopathic arthritis, so that their care can be planned for the long term from the outset.

Recognizing Particular Uveitis/Glaucoma Syndromes

Glaucomatocyclitic Crisis

Glaucomatocyclitic crisis (Posner-Schlossman syndrome) typically presents as an acute unilateral pressure elevation associated with mild inflammation. The patient's complaints relate to corneal edema – either blurring or halo vision. Pressures often reach the range of 40 to 55 mmHg, and the anterior chamber has a modest cellular response with little or no flare. The eye is not red. The usual error in diagnosis is to attribute the signs and symptoms to acute angle closure. Gonioscopy of both the involved eye and the opposite eye differentiates the two. Keratic precipitates may be absent initially but usually develop within a few days, when the anterior segment appearance resembles idiopathic iridocyclitis. A distinguishing feature is the lack of posterior synechiae in glaucomatocyclitic crisis.

Glaucomatocyclitic crises resolve spontaneously within a few weeks, with or without treatment. They often recur, and, although generally unilateral at any given episode, they may develop in both eyes. Both cupping and field loss may develop with recurrent or prolonged episodes. Patients with a typical history and typical physical findings do not need uveitis workups. Treat each episode with suppressants of aqueous humor formation. Corticosteroids are generally not necessary. Follow the guidelines on page 175 for the management of recurrent episodes of inflammation. Some individuals have elevated, albeit less elevated, pressure between episodes, which is managed by the routine guidelines for elevated IOP (Chapter 6).

Fuchs Heterochromic Iridocyclitis

This syndrome classically involves unilateral heterochromia (lighter on the involved side), inflammation, and cataract formation. Approximately 10% of cases are bilateral and may be difficult to diagnose. The cornea has characteristic small keratic precipitates that may be connected by fine filaments. The inflammation does not cause anterior or posterior synechiae (except at a rare Koeppe nodule), although it may be associated with mild anterior segment neovascularization. Pressure elevation develops in about 15% to 20% of patients. Because heterochromia, inflammation, and unilateral cataract formation usually precede pressure elevation, the condition often presents as elevated IOP in a unilaterally pseudophakic patient with mild inflammation. The inflammation associated with Fuchs heterochromic iridocyclitis is generally mild and does not improve with anti-inflammatory medication. Treatment with corticosteroids does not decrease the eye pressure. Medical treatment of the high pressure proceeds as described in the section for chronic uveitis and glaucoma, but treatment often fails to control the pressure.

Herpes Zoster or Simplex Uveitis with Elevated Pressure

Both herpes zoster ophthalmicus and herpes simplex keratouveitis are treated with antiviral agents. The routine guidelines for treating elevated IOP in uveitis apply to both conditions.

Phacolytic and/or Phacoantigenic Glaucoma

Lens protein leaks through the capsule of some mature and hypermature lenses. Macrophages ingest the protein and clog the trabecular meshwork, causing acute pressure elevations that may reach the range of 60 to 80 mmHg. The protein-laden macrophages are visible as large cells in the anterior chamber where they have been reported to glisten on slit-lamp examination (we have not found the glistening to be obvious). The patient's vision is poor. After obtaining an echographic screen of the fundus, we treat patients with no history of uveitis who have high pressure, large cells in the anterior chamber, and mature or hypermature cataracts as if they have phacolytic glaucoma and perform prompt cataract extraction with intraocular lens implantation.

Ciliary Body Rotation and Angle Closure Glaucoma

Inflammation of the ciliary body may cause the lens to move forward and close the angle by a posterior pushing mechanism (Figure 10-1). Symptoms include blurred vision (from increased myopia, corneal edema, or both) and photophobia. The central chamber has cells and flare. It is shallow and asymmetric to the opposite eye. Peripheral iridotomy does not resolve the angle closure, and the condition is treated with cycloplegia and corticosteroids. It is unusual among the uveitis/elevated pressure conditions in that angle closure is present at the onset and in that it is usually successfully treated.

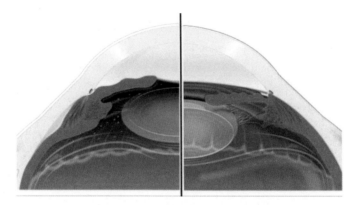

FIG 10-1. Ciliary body rotation and inflammation with angle closure, *left*; normal for comparison, *right*.

General Management of Patients with Elevated Pressure and Uveitis

The management of patients with elevated pressure associated with uveitis will be discussed as if patients could be divided into to three general categories:

- Patients with a single, short (less than 6 months) period of inflammation and high pressure; for example, idiopathic anterior uveitis, inflammation following surgery, or inflammation associated with blunt trauma
- Patients with recurrent episodes of inflammation and elevated pressure separated by intervals without inflammation, such as recurrent anterior uveitis and glaucomatocyclitic crises
- Patients with chronic uveitis associated with elevated pressure

In practice, even if a patient does fit neatly into one of these groups, it may not be apparent at presentation. We recommend treating new patients according to the guidelines for a single episode unless they clearly belong in one of the other groups.

For all three groups, there are two major constant recommendations that also apply to patients with uveitis who do not have elevated pressure: prevent or relieve pupillary block, and treat with as small a dose of corticosteroid as possible to control the inflammation.

Prevention or Relief of Pupillary Block

Posterior synechiae develop in inflamed eyes. If they entirely close the pupil, pupillary block ensues. Synechiae formation is related to the degree of inflammation and to the size and mobility of the pupil. Except for cases of glaucomatocyclitic crisis and Fuchs heterochromic iridocyclitis (which do not tend to develop posterior synechiae), cycloplegic drops are used in patients with iridocyclitis to prevent synechiae formation. If an eye is treated with chronic long-acting cycloplegics such as atropine, homatropine, or hyoscine, intermittent use of a mydriatic agent to move the pupil further decreases synechiae formation. Depending on the degree of inflammation, we suggest use of phenylephrine 2.5% once a day to once a week. To increase intraocular penetration and decrease systemic absorption, advise the patient either to close his or her lids or to use nasolacrimal obstruction for 5 minutes after the drops are instilled. Miotic drops exacerbate posterior synechiae formation and should be avoided.

If posterior synechiae are already present but there is no pupillary block, attempt to break as many as possible. Daily use of phenylephrine for 1 or 2 weeks in conjunction with either a short- or long-acting cycloplegic breaks many early adhesions.

When pupillary block and elevated pressure related to complete posterior synechiae develop in a patient with uveitis, it is reasonable to perform a laser iridotomy to decompress the eye. However, laser procedures may exacerbate inflammation, and the small holes achieved with laser treatment often close within a short time. We therefore recommend large and multiple iridotomies in patients with active inflammation. Surgical sector iridectomy may be necessary in such patients.

Use of Minimum Corticosteroids

Standard uveitis treatment includes the use of sufficient corticosteroids and cycloplegics to control the inflammation, with medications then tapered to as low a dosage as maintains control of inflammation. Inflamed eyes often have low pressures that rise as the inflammation is treated and the aqueous humor production rises. In addition to this indirect effect on pressure, corticosteroid use can also cause a direct pressure elevation in some individuals. It may be impossible to determine whether a patient's pressure rises because of increased aqueous humor production or because of decreased outflow from corticosteroid use, but provided the patient is being treated with as small a dose of steroid as possible (but enough to control the inflammation), the distinction is not clinically relevant. Topical and/or systemic non-steroidal anti-inflammatory drugs (NSAIDs) may be sufficient to control inflammation and should be tried whenever appropriate. We recommend that patients with more than intermittent need for topical steroid treatment be referred to a uveitis specialist if possible.

Management of a Single Episode of Inflammation and High Pressure

A patient who is expected to have a single episode of elevated pressure does not generally need a formal baseline exam. We examine the disc to determine whether the patient has evidence of cupping to suggest a chronic but unrecognized problem. We also examine the retinal periphery carefully because of the occasional association between peripheral retinal detachment, mild inflammation, and elevated pressure (Schwartz syndrome). At every follow-up visit we check the disc for hemorrhages or obviously increased cupping, but neither the inconvenience nor the expense of multiple visual fields and disc photographs or OCT seems warranted for most people. Not every patient has a brief and limited period of inflammation, and if the inflammation and elevated IOP persist for 6 months, then follow the guidelines for chronic uveitis (page 175).

We suggest arbitrary management guidelines in patients with an initial episode of inflammation and high pressure. We prefer to treat with topical medication only. Prostaglandin analogs are anecdotally reported to be contraindicated in the setting of active uveitis, though there is little evidence to suggest increased morbidity with their use and we use them. [1] Most patients tolerate short-term modest elevations of pressure. Most people also tolerate short-term marked elevations of pressure, but we do not assume that a patient's nerve can tolerate elevated pressure until the passage of time provides some information. We are reluctant to consider surgical intervention for what will probably be a temporary condition.

If the patient's history or physical examination suggests preexisting glaucoma, then we modify the following guidelines for target pressure as indicated by the state of the disc and field (Chapter 4).

IOP > 21 mmHg ≤ 30 mmHg

- Treat the inflammation.
- Taper corticosteroids as soon as reasonable.
- If pressure remains elevated after inflammation resolves and steroids are withdrawn, manage the patient as a glaucoma suspect.
- If inflammation and elevated pressure remain at 6 months, follow the guidelines for the management of chronic uveitis-associated elevated pressure (page 175).

IOP > 30 mmHg ≤ 40 mmHg

- Treat the inflammation.
- Taper corticosteroids as soon as possible.
- Treat with topical IOP-lowering medications (except miotics).
- Obtain baseline disc imaging and field examination.
- Follow at weekly intervals for 2 weeks and then at monthly intervals if the IOP does not fall below 30 mmHg. If the disc on any examination appears different from the baseline, use the management guidelines for patients with chronic uveitis associated with elevated pressure (page 175).
- If pressure remains elevated after the inflammation resolves and steroids are withdrawn, manage the patient as a glaucoma suspect due to ocular hypertension (Chapter 6).
- If inflammation and elevated pressure remain at 6 months, follow the guidelines for the management of chronic uveitis associated with elevated pressure.

IOP > 40 mmHg

- Treat the inflammation.
- Taper steroids as soon as possible.
- Treat with topical IOP-lowering medications; if needed use systemic carbonic anhydrase inhibitor to achieve an IOP below 40 mmHg.
- Obtain baseline disc imaging and field examination.
- Follow at weekly intervals for 2 weeks and then at monthly intervals if the IOP does not fall below 30 mmHg. If the disc on any examination appears different from the baseline, use the guidelines for management of chronic uveitis associated with elevated pressure (page 175).
- If the IOP cannot be lowered below 40 mmHg, consider surgery. If the angles are wide open, goniotomy or trabeculotomy may be effective. We avoid laser trabeculoplasty because it is ineffective and aggravates the inflammation. Filtration surgery on a uveitic eye has a low chance of success and unsuccessful surgery does not help the patient's condition. Glaucoma drainage devices (GDD, valved or non-valved) may be effective alternatives.[2-6] If the disc and field can be followed serially, we sometimes observe patients who have pressures in the 40 mmHg range until there is evidence of progression, although the risk of retinal venous occlusion in this setting is unknown and presumed to be increased compared to normotensive uveitis patients. We generally operate on patients with pressures above 50 mmHg;

we almost always recommend prompt surgery in individuals who have pulsatile central retinal arteries.

Management of Recurrent Episodes of Inflammation and Elevated Pressure Separated by Intervals Without Inflammation

When it is expected that the patient will have multiple episodes of inflammation and elevated pressure either by the diagnosis of a uveitic syndrome in which a recurrence is typical, or by history of multiple inflammatory episodes, establish a full baseline as described in Chapter 2 as soon as the currently active episode has quieted. Treat each episode's pressure as described for the initial single episode. After each bout of inflammation, repeat the visual field and disc examination and compare the findings to the baseline. If the patient develops progressive disc or field damage, then set a lower target pressure for treatment during subsequent episodes.

Some individuals who have recurrent inflammation with elevated IOP develop higher-than-normal pressures between episodes. Between episodes, use the follow-up schedule for glaucoma suspects due to ocular hypertension for such patients (Chapter 6). They may require treatment only during the episodes of inflammation and higher pressure if progressive damage only occurs at these times; however, if the pressure between episodes also produces harm, chronic treatment for glaucoma is required.

Management of Chronic Uveitis Associated with Elevated Pressure

Some types of uveitis, for example those associated with sarcoidosis and juvenile idiopathic arthritis, are chronic. In addition, apparently acute conditions may fail to resolve. After an arbitrary limit of 6 months, we assume that the uveitis will be chronic. When a person has elevated pressure and chronic uveitis, we attempt to lower the pressure even if there is no damage. In our experience, the risk of damage is sufficient to justify treatment in such cases. The principles of glaucoma care in patients with chronic uveitis are much the same as those for primary open angle glaucoma:

- Correct the correctable.
- Establish a baseline.
- Set a target pressure and treat to achieve the target.
- Continue to observe the patient to assess the stability of his or her condition.
- Modify target pressure and treatment as indicated.

Correction of the Correctable

Rule out or treat pupillary block. Control the inflammation, usually with corticosteroids, NSAIDs and cycloplegics. Refer to a uveitis or rheumatology specialist for consideration of steroid-sparing therapy. While the inflammation is being controlled, treat the pressure initially according to the guidelines listed under the single episode management section with the modification that patients with IOP > 21 mmHg but ≤ 30 mmHg are treated with topical agents.

Establishment of a Baseline

As soon as the inflammation is reasonably controlled, obtain baseline studies. Waiting until the inflammation is controlled usually increases the quality of the baseline studies. In a significantly inflamed eye, the nerve may be swollen and the cup falsely small. Photophobia, corneal edema, and inflammatory debris impede funduscopy and interfere with examination of the visual field. If the inflammation at the time of presentation is very mild, the vision is good, and the patient is comfortable, then start immediately to obtain baseline studies (Chapter 2).

Determination of a Target Pressure

When the patient has uveitis and elevated pressure on presentation, it is not possible to assume (as when dealing with asymptomatic pressure elevation) that the pressure has probably been at its level for a reasonably long period. Determine the target pressure as described in Chapter 4, but recognize that it is only an estimate, and that none of the clinical trial data to date provide useful information on the risk of glaucomatous conversion or progression.

Treatment to Achieve the Target Pressure

Treatment involves control of inflammation and suppression of aqueous humor formation with topical IOP-lowering agents. Avoid use of miotics because they exacerbate inflammation and promote posterior synechiae formation. Laser trabeculoplasty is not generally successful in inflammatory glaucoma, and surgery is both more difficult and less successful than in primary glaucoma.

We usually begin with a beta-blocker once or twice a day with the appropriate anti-inflammatory treatment. If the IOP remains higher than the target, we augment topical therapy as outlined in Chapter 4.

If cupping is mild and there is either no field loss or early loss, we usually add oral medication if the pressure is 40 mmHg or higher. If the cupping is moderate, and field loss, if present, is mild or moderate, we add oral medication at a pressure of about 32 mmHg or if the pressure has fallen less than 20%. If the cupping or field loss is severe, we prescribe systemic carbonic anhydrase inhibitors when the pressure is greater than about 26 mmHg or has decreased less than 30%.

We begin treatment with methazolamide 25 mg twice daily, and, if needed, increase to methazolamide 50 mg twice daily. If the pressure is still above the carbonic anhydrase inhibitor threshold and the patient tolerates methazolamide, we change the regimen to acetazolamide 250 mg four times daily or to Diamox Sequels twice daily. If the patient does not tolerate the medication, we discontinue it.

Follow-up

Because of the potential complications of uveitic glaucoma, we recommend using the follow-up schedule for severe glaucoma described in Chapter 5. *On each examination look* for and, if present, treat posterior synechiae and pupillary block. Perform gonioscopy frequently. Progressive PAS formation related to inflammatory debris generally dictates increased anti-inflammatory treatment and increases the probability that the pressure will rise. If the glaucoma is controlled surgically, then the follow-up schedule is dictated more by the uveitis management than the glaucoma management.

Modification of Target Pressure and Treatment

The principles of target pressure modification are described in Chapter 5. The usual practical question that arises in the chronic care of uveitic patients is if and when to move from medical to surgical management. Once it is reasonably certain that further visual field loss is likely with medical therapy alone, we usually recommend surgery. In our experience, laser surgery rarely helps, and we no longer perform trabeculoplasty in individuals with uveitis. The details of performing surgery on individuals with uveitis are discussed in standard surgery texts.

Standard filtering procedures augmented with anti-fibrotic agents rarely offer long-term IOP control in active uveitis, though in select patients, especially those who have received intravitreal steroid implants, filtering procedures are a reasonable option.[2] Circumferential or partial angle surgery from a temporal approach may lower the IOP without compromising future surgical options, especially if the history suggests a large steroid-induced component contributing to the IOP elevation. [3,4]

When angle surgery cannot be performed, we almost always proceed with GDD placement. GDDs offer good short- and long-term outcomes, comparable to that of primary open angle glaucoma in some studies. [5,6] A valved device may decrease the risk of hypotony compared to non-valved devices. Before surgery, we consult with a uveitis specialist to help manage the ocular inflammation.

Common Problems in the Care of Chronic Uveitis Associated with Elevated Pressure

Although it is easy to offer guidelines for the care of patients with chronic uveitis associated with elevated pressure, in practice it can be difficult to decide the best course for an individual patient. Two common problems that arise in the management of these patients are the following:

- Steroid-related pressure elevation
- Cataract interference with visual fields and fundus visualization

Steroid-Related Pressure Elevation

As noted, treating with as small a dose of steroid as possible to control the inflammation is one of the general guides for managing glaucoma and uveitis. If a patient appears to have a significant pressure elevation that might be steroid related, the question sometimes arises of whether to change to a different drug, for example an antimetabolite or biologic agent, for control of the uveitis. Usually a patient in whom this course is considered has bilateral uveitis that corticosteroids can control, but also has glaucoma related to the steroid treatment. We refer these patients to a uveitis specialist for consultation.

Cataract Interference

When cataract precludes adequate fundus evaluation and field examination in a patient with chronic uveitis and glaucoma, our treatment recommendation depends on the type of uveitis and the degree of pressure elevation. We use a routine surgical approach in patients with herpetic eye disease, glaucomatocyclitic crisis and Fuchs heterochromic iridocyclitis when the patient considers his or her disability sufficient to warrant the risk of surgery. When cataract surgery is elected in individuals with idiopathic chronic uveitis or in chronic uveitis associated with sarcoidosis, we perform cataract extraction and intraocular lens implantation after the eye is quiet for at least 6 months. Pars plana lensectomy with concurrent vitrectomy is usually performed in children and young adults with juvenile idiopathic arthritis, who are often left aphakic.

References

1. Horsley MB, Chen TC. The use of prostaglandin analogs in the uveitic patient. Seminars in Ophthalmology. 2011 Jul-Sep;26(4-5):285-9.

2. Bollinger K, Kim J, Lowder CY, Kaiser PK, Smith SD. Intraocular pressure outcome of patients with fluocinolone acetonide intravitreal implant for noninfectious uveitis. Ophthalmology. 2011 Oct;118(10):1927-31.

3. Anton A, Heinzelmann S, Neß T, Lübke J, Neuburger M, Jordan JF, Wecker T. Trabeculectomy ab interno with the Trabectome® as a therapeutic option for uveitic secondary glaucoma. Graefe's Archives for Clinical and Experimental Ophthalmology. 2015 Nov;253(11):1973-8.

4. Shimizu A, Maruyama K, Yokoyama Y, Tsuda S, Ryu M, Nakazawa T. Characteristics of uveitic glaucoma and evaluation of its surgical treatment. Journal of Clinical Ophthalmology. 2014 Nov 26;8:2383-9.

5. Da Mata A, Burk SE, Netland PA, Baltatzis S, Christen W, Foster CS. Management of uveitic glaucoma with Ahmed glaucoma valve implantation. Ophthalmology. 1999 Nov;106(11):2168-72.

6. Rachmiel R, Trope GE, Buys YM, Flanagan JG, Chipman ML. Ahmed glaucoma valve implantation in uveitic glaucoma versus open angle glaucoma patients. Canadian Journal of Ophthalmology. 2008 Aug;43(4):462-7.

11 ELEVATED PRESSURE IN SURGICAL AND NONSURGICAL TRAUMA

With a few exceptions, the mechanisms of elevated pressure after intraocular surgery, accidental penetrating trauma, and blunt trauma are the same. Evaluation and management of high pressure after trauma follow four straightforward steps:

- Determine the probable mechanism(s) of the pressure elevation.
- Manage the emergent and treatable causes of elevated intraocular pressure (IOP) – infection and angle closure.
- Manage residual pressure elevation as the eye recovers.
- Proceed to chronic care of elevated IOP if the pressure elevation does not resolve.

After describing the mechanisms of elevated pressure after trauma, we present algorithms for the evaluation of patients with high pressure in two prototype situations: high pressure following intraocular surgery and high pressure following blunt trauma. For simplicity, we refer to nonsurgical injury as accidental, regardless of whether the injury was purposeful, and assume that blunt trauma has not caused scleral rupture. Ruptured globes and eyes that have sustained penetrating accidental trauma generally have low pressure initially. If the pressure becomes elevated after surgical repair, they are included in the category of postoperative pressure elevation.

Most high pressures resolve within a few weeks after surgery or other trauma. If the pressure remains elevated after the first month, re-evaluate the patient for one of the causes of late pressure elevation. If no reversible cause is found and the pressure is still high after 3 months, follow the guides for routine management of chronic high pressure: establish a baseline, decide if treatment is indicated and, if it is, set a target pressure, treat to achieve the target, continue to observe the patient, and modify the target and treatment if indicated.

Identifying the Mechanisms of Elevated Pressure in Penetrating and Nonpenetrating Trauma

Table 11-1 summarizes the major causes of IOP elevation after surgical trauma and accidental nonpenetrating trauma. Several conditions may occur concurrently.

Early Mechanisms of Pressure Elevation

Acute infection. Endophthalmitis may cause pressure elevation, perhaps because inflammatory debris blocks aqueous outflow. Once appropriate antimicrobial treatment is begun, examine the eye regularly to identify other mechanisms of pressure elevation.

Inflammation. Inflammation raises eye pressure by the mechanisms discussed in Chapter 10. In addition to nonspecific inflammation related to trauma, retained lens material incites inflammation that generally persists until the lens material is resorbed, removed, or encapsulated. Inflammation related to lens material may explode, as does phacoantigenic endophthalmitis, or it may smolder, as does most inflammation from retained lens cortex after cataract surgery. An intact but subluxed or dislocated lens does not generally cause inflammation.

TABLE 11-1. Major Causes of Elevated Pressure after Trauma

Acute causes of elevated IOP	Surgical trauma	Blunt trauma
Infection	x	
Inflammation	x	x
Pupillary block	x	x
Other types of angle closure	x	x
Hyphema	x	x
Residual viscoelastic material	x	
Direct damage to the outflow system	x	x
Late causes of elevated IOP		
Chronic infection	x	
Steroid-induced elevated IOP	x	x
Peripheral anterior synechiae	x	x
Ghost cell and hemolytic glaucoma	x	x
Angle trauma and dysfunction	x	x
Epithelial ingrowth	x	

Pupillary block. Pupillary block may be seen early or it may develop, with or without symptoms, sometime after surgery or injury. Pupillary block rarely develops in an eye with a patent peripheral iridotomy. It is particularly common in eyes with anterior chamber lenses and no iridotomy.

Adhesions of the iris to the vitreous face, lens, or lens implant may block passage of aqueous humor toward or through the pupil. Figure 11-1 illustrates some variants on pupillary block that may develop after surgical or accidental trauma. If only the pupil margin is adherent to underlying structures, the iris leaf bows forward, giving a typical iris bombé appearance (bulging of the iris further anterior than the pupil plane) as posterior chamber pressure increases. If much of the posterior iris surface is adherent, only the mobile peripheral iris may protrude forward, and iris bombé may be apparent only in the peripheral anterior chamber. Before complete blockage develops, the bulging peripheral iris may crowd the angle without closing it and producing an elevated pressure. Peripheral iris bulge without high IOP should be treated if noted.

Lens subluxation, which may occur from blunt trauma, causes relative pupillary block related to forward movement of the lens and may, in combination with vitreous gel, cause pupillary block.

Posterior pushing angle closure. In the early postoperative or post-traumatic period, angle closure with elevated pressure may develop in several ways other than pupillary block. For discussion, we divide these into ciliary block and forward rotation of the iris-lens diaphragm. This distinction is arbitrary and the underlying pathophysiologic mechanism is often unclear.

Ciliary block. Ciliary block, also known as vitreous block, malignant glaucoma and aqueous misdirection, is a condition in which aqueous humor presumably does not freely enter the posterior chamber because of relative resistance somewhere in the zonular/capsular/hyaloid face junction. The central anterior chamber is shallow because the lens or vitreous face is pushed forward, and peripheral iridotomy neither prevents nor resolves the angle closure. Ciliary block most typically occurs in an eye with a small anterior segment and an anatomically narrow angle. The precise mechanism of ciliary block is not well-understood, but a model that explains the central chamber shallowing and its resolution with cycloplegia is illustrated in Figure 11-2. [1]

Forward rotation of the iris-lens diaphragm. Ciliary body inflammation, ciliary body or suprachoroidal hemorrhage, and scleral buckling may each cause the ciliary body to rotate inward around its attachment to the scleral spur. This moves the iris-lens diaphragm forward (Figures 10-1, 11-6, and 11-8). The angle closure that results does not generally resolve after iridotomy, although the angle may widen with cycloplegia. Suprachoroidal hemorrhage also acutely raises the IOP by a mass effect, but after compensatory exit of aqueous humor the eye returns to equilibrium; a nonexpanding mass does not cause persistent elevated pressure in the absence of angle closure.

Hyphema. Blood in the anterior chamber may raise the pressure in at least two ways. A clot that spans the pupil will cause pupillary block (Figures 11-1 D and 11-3). As serum and aqueous humor exit through the meshwork, the posterior chamber expands because the aqueous humor cannot pass the pupil. The iris thus moves forward to close the angle while the red cells become compacted. Even in the absence of pupillary block, red blood cells may block the trabecular meshwork. The red cells of patients with sickle cell trait or sickle cell disease may sickle in the anterior chamber and, being inflexible, block outflow for longer than nonsickled cells. Vitreous hemorrhage without hyphema does not cause elevated IOP acutely, although blood in the vitreous cavity may later cause both ghost cell and hemolytic glaucoma (discussed in a later section).

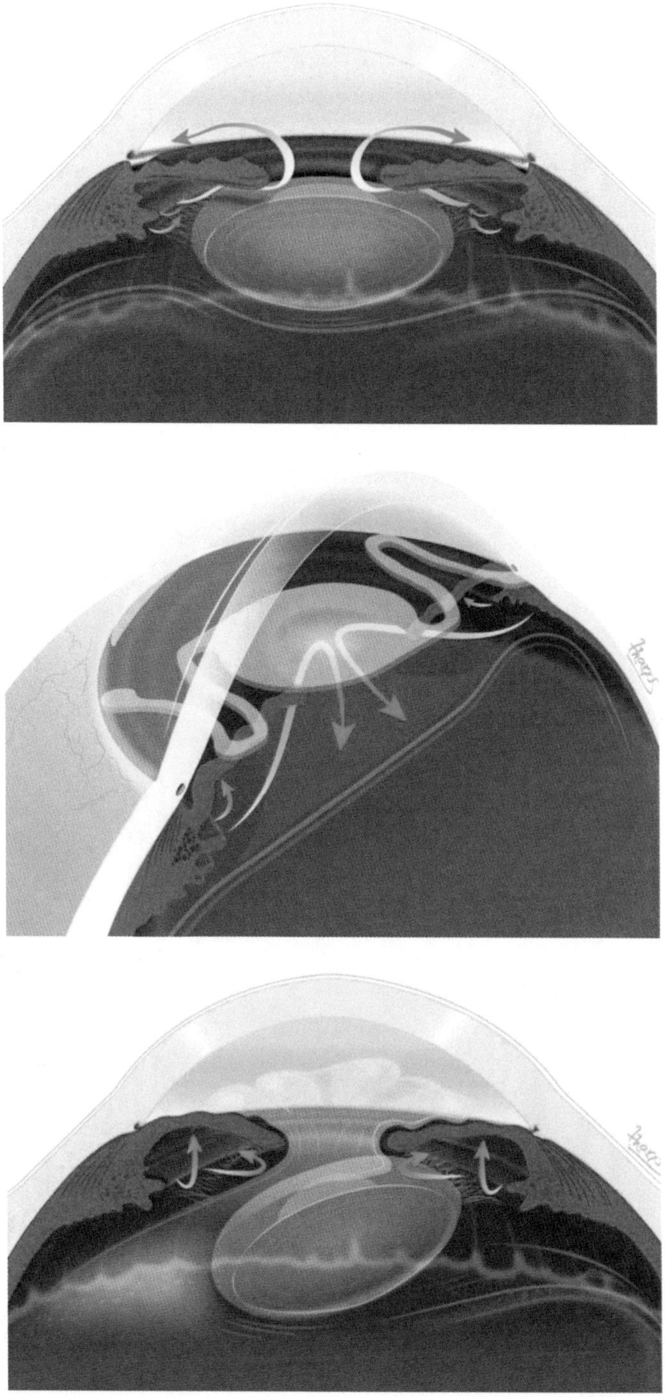

A

B

C

FIG. 11-1. Variations on pupillary block after trauma. **A**. Normal aqueous humor flow. **B**. Anterior chamber intraocular lens causing pupillary block **C**. Herniated vitreous humor causing pupillary block (*continued on next page*).

D

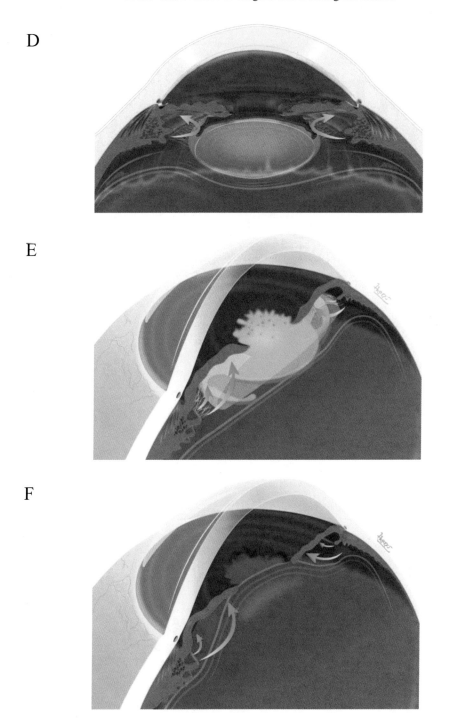

E

F

FIG 11-1 (continued). Variations on pupillary block after trauma. **D**. Collar button clot causing pupillary block. **E**. Synechiae to the lens causing pupillary block. **F**. Synechiae to the vitreous face causing pupillary block.

A

B

C

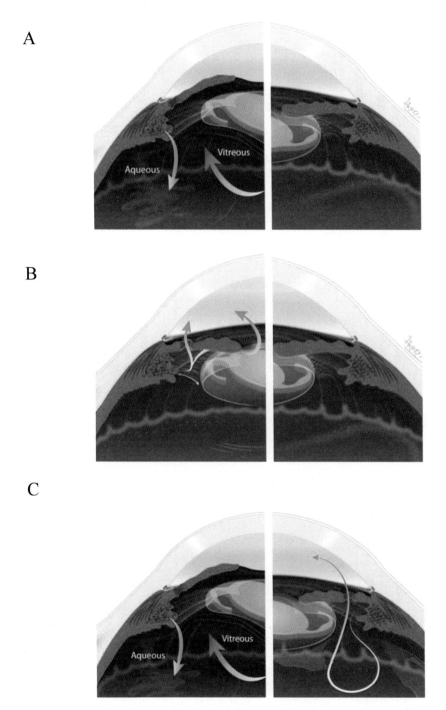

FIG. 11-2 **A.** Ciliary block, *left*; normal for comparison, *right*. The lens moves forward, pressing the iris and shallowing the central chamber. Aqueous humor flows backward into the vitreous body pushing the vitreous face forward. **B.** Resolution of ciliary block after atropine administration, *left*; normal for comparison, *right*. Atropine pulls the lens implant back. The iris falls back, and aqueous humor flows into the anterior chamber. **C.** Ciliary block, *left*; resolution of ciliary block after anterior hyaloidectomy/vitrectomy, zonulectomy, and iridectomy, *right*. The creation of a unicameral eye is the definitive surgical treatment of ciliary block refractory to medical treatment.

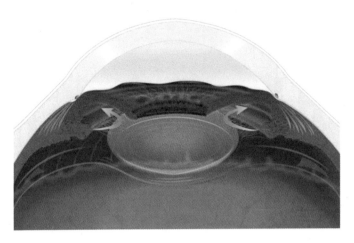

FIG. 11-3. Small clot causing pupillary block by sticking the pupillary border to the lens. See also Figure 11-1D.

Viscoelastic material in the eye. Mechanical blockage of the trabecular meshwork by viscoelastic material can raise the pressure until the substance dissolves. Dissolution generally occurs within 48 hours.

Direct trauma to the outflow system. Blunt ocular trauma indents the eye at the point of impact, transiently raising the IOP and stretching the intraocular structures and the ocular coat (Figure 11-4). Ciliary muscle rupture results in "angle recession" and hyphema. Stretching of the ocular coat causes microshredding of the trabecular meshwork and flap tears in the meshwork. Ciliary muscle and trabecular meshwork damage lead to swelling (early) and scarring (late), which impair aqueous humor outflow and result in high pressure. A large limbal cataract incision may likewise damage the trabecular meshwork and the collector channels, though this is rarely seen nowadays.

A

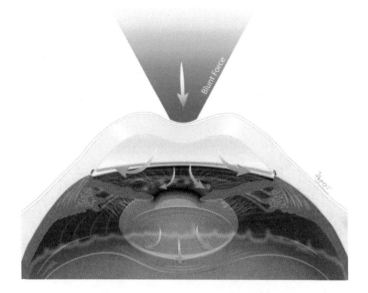

B

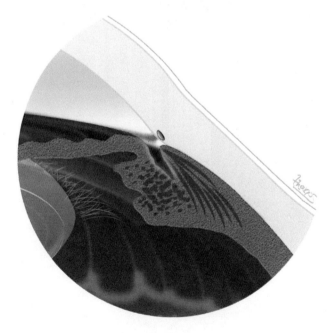

FIG. 11-4. Blunt ocular trauma. **A.** (*this page*) Force is transmitted to all of the intraocular structures. **B.** A tear between layers of the ciliary muscle produces an angle recession. **C.** (*next page*) A flap tear in the face of the trabecular meshwork. **D.** A tear in the zonular ring may allow vitreous body herniation.

C

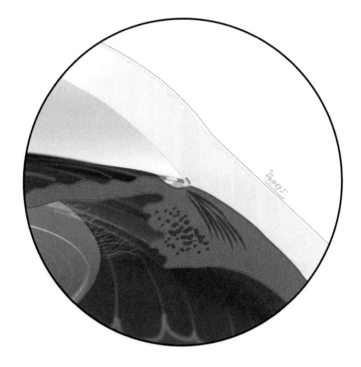

D

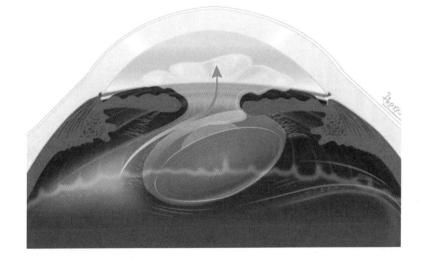

Later Causes of Elevated Pressure

Chronic infection. Subacute and chronic infection may elude diagnosis for months. The most common organism to cause low-grade infection after eye surgery is *Propionibacterium acnes*, which sometimes causes pressure elevations associated with smoldering inflammation.

Corticosteroid-induced pressure elevation. Corticosteroids directly affect IOP by decreasing the ease of aqueous humor outflow. They may indirectly raise pressure in inflamed eyes by decreasing inflammation, thereby increasing aqueous humor production. After uncomplicated surgery or mild trauma, corticosteroids can generally be discontinued if they are suspected of elevating the pressure. Following complicated surgery or significant trauma associated both with outflow system damage and lingering inflammation requiring continued corticosteroid use, it may be difficult to determine the precise contribution of corticosteroids to high pressure.

Blood-induced elevated IOP. Blood enters the vitreous cavity in two ways: a hyphema may move backward through a rent in the zonule-posterior capsule diaphragm, or the patient may have a hemorrhage from a posterior structure directly into the vitreous cavity. Blood in the vitreous cavity resorbs slowly. Red cells may degenerate, and, if degenerated cells or their breakdown products move into the anterior chamber, may cause either ghost cell glaucoma or hemolytic glaucoma. The convention is to refer to these conditions as "glaucoma" even if optic damage is not demonstrated.

Ghost cell glaucoma. Ghost cells are degenerated red blood cells, which have become spherical rather than disc-shaped and appear tan or khaki-colored. Like sickled cells, they are inflexible and may block the trabecular meshwork and increase resistance to outflow.

Hemolytic glaucoma. Fragments of hemolyzed red cells and macrophages laden with blood breakdown products may block the trabecular meshwork and cause hemolytic glaucoma. The cells in the anterior chamber are red.

Angle closure –

Peripheral anterior synechiae. Peripheral anterior synechiae (PAS) develop from the healing of ruptures in the trabecular meshwork and face of the ciliary body, from healing of an incision, or from prolonged contact between the iris and the trabecular meshwork, especially in an inflamed eye. They directly block outflow and raise outflow pressure in proportion to the extent of meshwork covered.

Epithelial ingrowth. When epithelial cells grow through a limbal or corneal wound, they first cover the posterior cornea and the anterior chamber angle, and the epithelial sheet then pulls the iris up over the meshwork.

Angle trauma and dysfunction. Blunt ocular trauma may produce immediate and persistent pressure elevation, or may be followed by normal pressure for many months, years or decades before the pressure increases. An acute pressure elevation may not occur, even in the presence of substantial outflow system damage, because of other effects of trauma such as decreased aqueous humor production. Thus a history of normal pressure in the early stages after an injury does not rule out subsequent pressure elevation related to trabecular meshwork damage. Chronic inflammation and secondary pigment dispersion, which sometimes result from a poorly positioned/mobile intraocular lens, may also result in outflow system damage.

Evaluating the Patient

History

Preexisting ocular disease. If the condition of the patient's eye before surgery or accidental injury is not known, try to determine by history the preexisting vision and question the patient regarding previous glaucoma. In the absence of better information, the status of the opposite eye indicates the likely previous status of the involved eye.

Pain. Severe pain generally accompanies acute endophthalmitis and suprachoroidal hemorrhage.

Hematologic history. Determine whether the patient has any known hematologic conditions, particularly a bleeding disorder or sickle hemoglobinopathy.

Operative history. If the media are clear, the physical exam – revealing what *is* present rather than what *might be* present – is more useful than operative history. However, if blood, corneal edema or inflammatory debris obscures the view, the operative history may suggest diagnostic possibilities. For example, if the capsule ruptured during a phacoemulsification, both nucleus and cortex may be present within the eye. Vitreous loss does not itself increase the IOP, but it is usually associated with additional manipulation and inflammation. If no peripheral iridectomy was performed, particularly if an anterior chamber lens was inserted, consider pupillary block. Use of intravitreal gas or silicone oil tamponade may result in angle closure.

Vision

Profoundly decreased vision (worse than hand motion) in the absence of hyphema suggests either infection or significant posterior segment injury.

Pupillary Examination

Test for an afferent defect and record the findings. The consensual pupil response (Marcus-Gunn sign) is helpful if the response of the pupil in the injured eye is indeterminate.

External Examination

Periorbital edema and marked conjunctival injection suggest a possible infection.

Slit Lamp Examination

Anterior chamber. Hypopyon or marked inflammation, particularly if inflammation involves the vitreous body, strongly suggests infection. Hyphema following blunt trauma is evidence of a tear in the uveal tissue of the angle and indicates likely trabecular meshwork damage. The clinician should examine the eye specifically with a narrow beam to see if the peripheral iris is in contact with the peripheral cornea, in which case the angle is obviously closed, or if a visible space extends as far to the peripheral anterior chamber as can be seen. If the peripheral anterior chamber is shallow or if the angle appears to be closed, determine if the central chamber is shallow.

Iris. If iris bombé is present, study the pupil to see if blood, vitreous humor, fibrin, or a fibrous adhesion is blocking the passage of aqueous humor. Note if there is a peripheral iridotomy or iridodialysis and, if one is present, whether it appears to be patent or clogged, for example, with vitreous humor. If the patient is pseudophakic, inspect for transillumination defects that outline the optic or haptics of the intraocular lens implant which may suggest components of the uveitis-glaucoma-hyphema (UGH) syndrome (Figure 11-7).

Lens. Phacodonesis suggests either a history of trauma or pseudoexfoliation. If the patient is pseudophakic, note any asymmetry in the distance between the iris border and the anterior lens surface at opposite poles, which may hint at a tilted, subluxed or decentered implant and UGH syndrome. Typically, an implant positioned in the anterior chamber or the sulcus is more likely to result in UGH syndrome than an implant positioned in the intracapsular space.

Gonioscopy

Iris bombé indicates pupillary block and may preclude gonioscopy until after relief of the block. If the iris does not show bombé, and if the view is adequate, perform gonioscopy to rule out angle closure.

Funduscopy

Vitreous inflammation suggests infection or lens material in the vitreous. If the eye is inflamed and the capsule was broken, look carefully for retained lens material.

Vitreous blood indicates that either a hyphema moved backward through a rent in the zonule-posterior capsule diaphragm or that the patient had a hemorrhage directly into the vitreous. Unless the cause of vitreous blood is clear, evaluate the patient for evidence of unrecognized penetrating injury (as with a retrobulbar needle) despite the usual association of hypotony with penetration. Look for a choroidal detachment, which in an eye with high pressure, usually indicates suprachoroidal hemorrhage.

Ancillary Testing and Laboratory Examination

If possible, echography should be performed in patients who have unexplained angle closure or in patients whose fundi cannot be visualized.

We obtain a sickle preparation for a patient of African or Afro-Caribbean descent with a hyphema and elevated pressure; we also obtain a sickle preparation for any patient who has a hyphema without pupillary block and an unexplained pressure elevation that is disproportionate to the amount of blood. Hemoglobin S is most common among patients known to be of African descent, but it occurs in all races.

Diagnosis and Management of High Pressure After Surgical and Accidental Trauma

We describe our diagnostic approach to elevated pressure in these prototypical situations: immediately after intraocular surgery, weeks to a few months following surgery, and promptly following blunt trauma.

Elevated IOP Early After Intraocular Surgery

Chart 11-1 summarizes the diagnosis of high pressure in the early postoperative period after intraocular surgery.

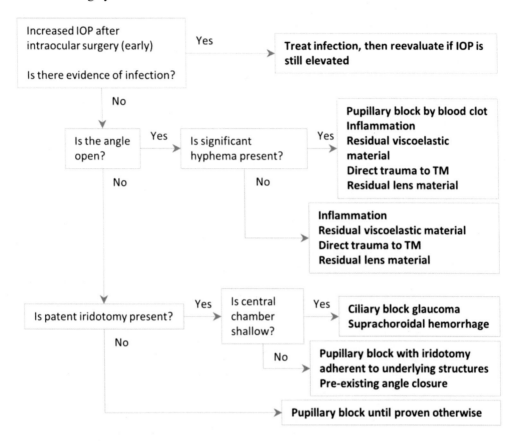

CHART 11-1. Diagnosis of high pressure in early postoperative period after intraocular surgery. Key – TM (trabecular meshwork).

Early elevated IOP – significant inflammation, other evidence of possible infection. Acute postoperative intraocular infection causes impressive pain, decreased vision, and both intraocular and extraocular inflammation. The infection, not the pressure, requires emergent care. Treat the pressure elevation according to the guidelines in Chapter 10 for a single episode of inflammation. If the pressure remains elevated after the infection has been treated appropriately, manage it like any other postoperative pressure elevation.

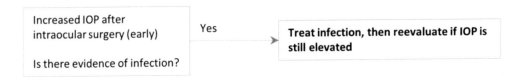

Early elevated IOP – open angle. Causes of elevated pressure with an open angle include sterile inflammation, retained lens material, residual viscoelastic material, hyphema, and direct trauma to the outflow mechanism from the surgical incision. Retained nuclear material should generally be removed surgically, but the other possibilities are treated by the guidelines for treatment of inflammation and elevated pressure described in Chapter 10. If there is a total hyphema, refer to page 207.

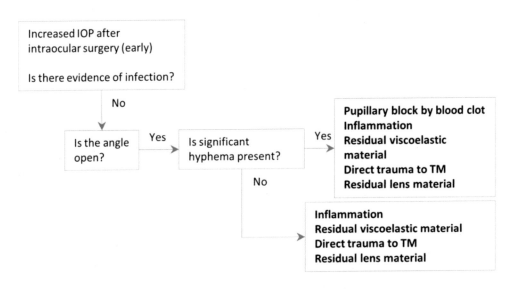

Early elevated IOP – closed angle. Angle closure that develops in the immediate postoperative period is usually obvious on slit lamp examination. Pupillary block caused by adhesions of the pupil margin to the underlying intraocular lens, vitreous, or capsule, or by apposition of the pupil to an overlying anterior chamber lens is the most common cause of early angle closure. Ciliary block accounts for a smaller number of closure cases. It is usually possible to distinguish between the two conditions at presentation. In an eye with pupillary block, the central chamber is of normal depth and the iris bulges forward from the pupil plane. In cases of ciliary block, the central anterior chamber is shallow or flat (Figure 11-5).

Pupillary block. Perform a laser peripheral iridotomy promptly if the cornea is sufficiently clear. In a pseudophakic patient, it may be necessary to perform the iridotomy in the midsection or even near the pupil because of iridocorneal touch peripherally. If so, perform a second iridotomy in the periphery after the bombé is relieved if inflammation persists and the more central opening is draped on a posterior structure in such a way that it might become closed by a new adhesion.

If the view is inadequate or if a laser is not immediately available, pupillary dilation will, in many cases, break fresh synechiae and relieve pupillary block. The use of phenylephrine to pull actively on the pupil is important, since simple paralysis of the pupil with a cycloplegic agent will not tug on adhesions. Even if the blockage is lysed to produce a clear channel, perform a prompt laser peripheral iridotomy. If there are peripheral anterior synechiae or if elevated pressure persists after relief of the pupillary block, manage the patient's condition according to the guidelines in Chapter 9 (pages 165-166) for chronic care after acute angle closure.

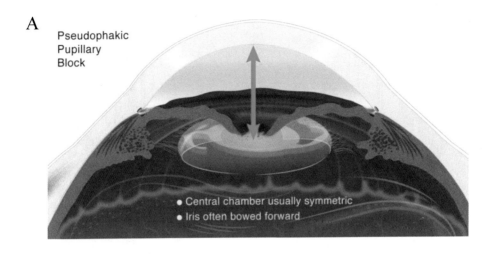

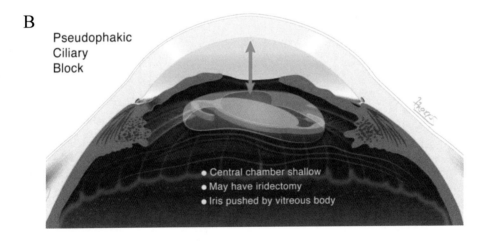

FIG. 11-5. Comparison of the usual presentations of pseudophakic pupillary block and pseudophakic ciliary block. **A.** In pseudophakic pupillary block, the central chamber is symmetric with fellow eye and peripheral iris bows forward in a bombé configuration. The situation is resolved by performing an iridotomy. **B.** In pseudophakic ciliary block the central chamber is shallow despite a patent iridotomy. The iris-lens diaphragm is pushed forward by the vitreous face.

Ciliary block. When managing presumed ciliary block after intraocular surgery, we recommend following several courses simultaneously to lower the pressure and reverse the mechanisms of angle closure. If the patient does not have a patent iridotomy, perform a laser iridotomy as soon as possible to remove the pupillary block element that is always present if the lens or implant is forward. Treat the eye with a strong cycloplegic agent and suppressants of aqueous humor formation to help maintain a low pressure when the underlying process is interrupted, but do not use miotics. In a pseudophakic patient, disrupt the posterior capsule and the anterior hyaloid face with the yttrium-aluminum-garnet (YAG) laser if possible. If the fundus is not visible, obtain an echographic exam to rule out a posterior lesion, such as suprachoroidal hemorrhage. If these measures do not resolve the ciliary block within a few hours, we refer the patient to a vitreous surgeon for pars plana vitrectomy, hyaloidectomy and iridectomy for creation of a unicameral eye (see box).

Timetable for Ciliary Block Management after Intraocular Surgery	
Immediate (not all these can be done at the same time, but they should all proceed as promptly as possible)	Laser peripheral iridotomy
	Atropine 1%, 1 drop q5 minutes x 3
	Topical IOP-lowering medications
	Acetazolamide 500 mg PO (if needed)
	YAG laser disruption of posterior capsule (if pseudophakic)
Before surgery (if fundus cannot be seen)	Echography to rule out posterior lesions
Within several hours (if block does not resolve)	Refer to vitreous surgeon for pars plana vitrectomy, hyaloidectomy, and iridectomy

Other causes. Suprachoroidal hemorrhage sometimes causes angle closure, probably by rotating the ciliary body forward, as illustrated in Figure 11-6. Laser iridotomy is contraindicated if the iris is too close to the cornea or if the retina/choroid is immediately behind the iris. Treat the patient with cycloplegics and topical/systemic IOP-lowering medications. The pressure usually decreases, and the posterior segment findings rather than the IOP usually guide management decisions. If the angle does not open and the pressure does not fall, the blood may be surgically drained.

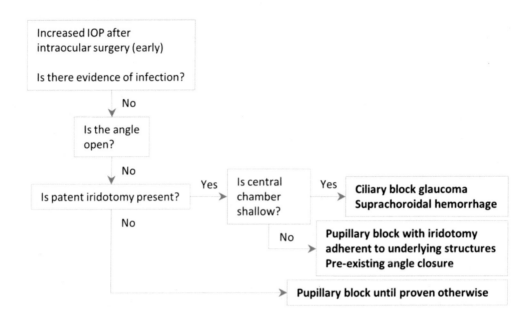

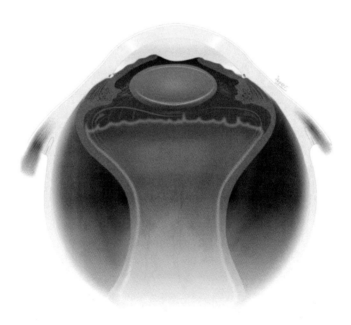

FIG. 11-6. Suprachoroidal hemorrhage causing forward rotation of the iris and ciliary body with angle closure.

Elevated IOP Later After Intraocular Surgery

Chart 11-2 summarizes the diagnostic steps for a patient who has either persistent or newly noted elevated pressure several weeks or months after intraocular surgery. The primary division, into eyes with cells in the anterior chamber and eyes without cells, serves to divide eyes that have not stabilized postoperatively from eyes that have stabilized. When the eye is free of inflammation (without use of corticosteroids) and any active pupillary block is relieved by iridotomy, the guidelines for treating any chronic elevated IOP also apply to the postoperative eye.

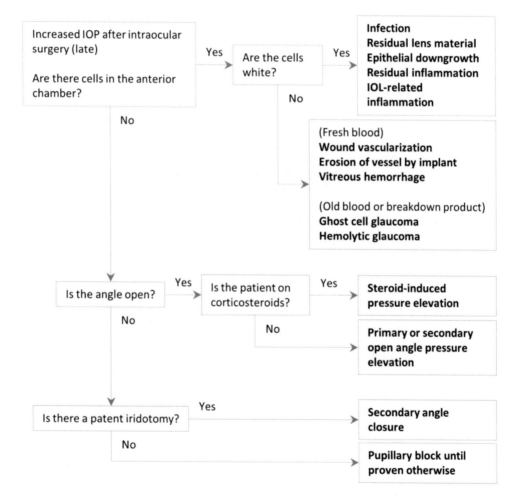

CHART 11-2. Diagnosis of high pressure in late postoperative period after intraocular surgery. Key – IOL (intraocular lens implant), IOP (intraocular pressure).

Later elevated IOP – cells in the anterior chamber. Inflammatory cells, red cells, denatured red cells, and epithelial cells may be found in the anterior chambers of eyes with postoperative pressure elevation. The cells usually appear either white or colored. Even if the color is not obvious, associated signs allow the clinician to distinguish among the various likely conditions in this setting. Always perform gonioscopy to rule out concurrent angle closure.

Persistent inflammation develops only rarely after intraocular surgery and often indicates a significant problem. The specifically treatable condition – and thus the most important to diagnose – is low-grade infection.

White cells –

Infection. Low-grade smoldering infection may cause secondary inflammation and high pressure. Anterior chamber tap and culture, if positive, confirms this diagnosis. However, culture results may be negative in the most commonly-recognized situation, that of *Propionibacterium acnes* infection, because the bacterium may be sequestered in residual cortex and capsule. Treatment depends on the organism being found or suspected and often includes removal of residual lens and capsule. As with acute endophthalmitis after treatment, any of the other postoperative mechanisms of elevated pressure may also develop.

Residual lens material. Persistent high pressure related to residual cortex raises therapeutic, not diagnostic problems in the late period. We suggest surgical removal of residual lens material as soon as possible, provided that this can be done safely. If high pressure persists, use the guides for IOP management discussed in Chapter 10 (page 166). If the patient has such significant glaucomatous damage that further loss is likely to cause significant visual impairment, we do simultaneous cortex removal and glaucoma surgery.

Epithelial ingrowth. A cellular membrane with an obvious line on the posterior cornea, large clumps of cells in the anterior segment, and very high IOP characterize epithelial ingrowth. If epithelial ingrowth is suspected, argon or diode laser application may help to make a diagnosis because epithelial cells turn white when coagulated. This test is not always easy to interpret, particularly in a blue-eyed individual.

The laser setting and technique are as follows:

- Large spots (200 microns)
- Long duration (0.5 second)
- Low energy (100 to 400 mW)

Apply treatment to the iris in the area of presumed ingrowth. Increase energy from 100 mW gradually until the iris surface contracts. If the iris surface chars, decrease energy since a charred epithelial membrane closely resembles a charred normal iris surface. If the treated area turns white, then use laser burns to determine the extent of involvement.

The surgical treatment of epithelial ingrowth is described in surgical texts.

Intraocular lens (IOL)-related inflammation. Inflammation related to lens implants may develop if a lens is mobile or not ideally positioned. An implant that is positioned outside the intracapsular space, such as in the anterior chamber or in the ciliary sulcus, or a mobile intracapsular implant related to zonulopathy, results in inflammation more frequently than an immobile intracapsular implant (Figure 11-7). The following signs and symptoms support this diagnosis:

- Tenderness of the limbus over the haptics of the lens without tenderness of the globe between the haptics.
- Shifting position of an anterior chamber IOL on serial examinations.
- Iris tucking or ciliary body indentation visible by gonioscopy.
- Iris transillumination defects outlining the IOL haptics/optic.

The initial treatment of inflammation related to implants follows the routine uveitis guides (Chapter 10). If the inflammation and elevated pressure do not resolve, the implant should generally be removed.

A

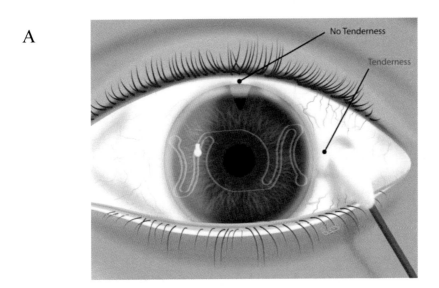

B

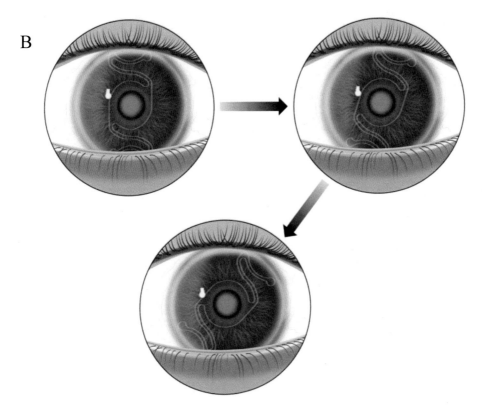

FIG. 11-7. Intraocular lens (IOL)-related inflammation. **A.** Limbal tenderness over the haptic in the setting of an anterior chamber intraocular lens. **B.** Shifting positions of an IOL on serial examinations indicate an improperly-sized lens. *(continued next page)*

202

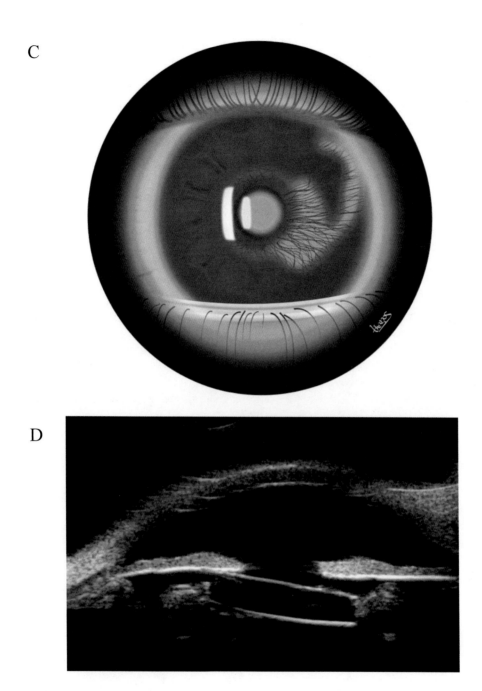

FIG. 11-7 (continued). Intraocular lens (IOL)-related inflammation. **C.** Iris transillumination defect outlining IOL haptic. **D.** High-resolution anterior segment ultrasound demonstrating a Soemmering's ring tilting a sulcus-positioned IOL and causing iris chafing.

Colored cells. Most hyphemas clear from the anterior chamber within the early postoperative period. Fresh blood thus indicates recurrent hemorrhage. Colored cells that do not resemble fresh blood indicate either ghost cell or hemolytic glaucoma. Both of these conditions develop when blood in the vitreous cavity denatures and then moves into the anterior chamber through a broken capsular-zonular diaphragm.

Fresh hemorrhage. Hyphema without vitreous hemorrhage and without neovascularization of the iris usually indicates either vascularization of the surgical wound or erosion of a uveal vessel by an implant. Diagnosis may be difficult and is sometimes made only after several gonioscopic examinations reveal a very localized clot beneath which a vascular nubbin is seen after the clot resolves. Definitive management of these conditions is discussed in standard surgical texts. The clinician should manage each episode of acute pressure elevation associated with hyphema following the guidelines in Chapter 10 for recurrent episodes of elevated pressure from inflammation. This includes use of corticosteroids to retard synechiae formation while the hemorrhage resorbs.

Ghost cell glaucoma. Tan or khaki-colored cells in the anterior chamber of a patient with elevated IOP who has had blood in the vitreous cavity indicate ghost cell glaucoma. The condition is self-limited. Adjust the follow-up frequency and ocular hypotensive therapy using the guides in Chapter 10 for a single episode of inflammation (page 173-175), but do not use corticosteroids. If the pressure does not fall below 32 mmHg, we generally perform both a vitrectomy and an anterior chamber washout.

Hemolytic glaucoma. The cells in the anterior chamber are red. Treatment is the same as that of ghost cell glaucoma.

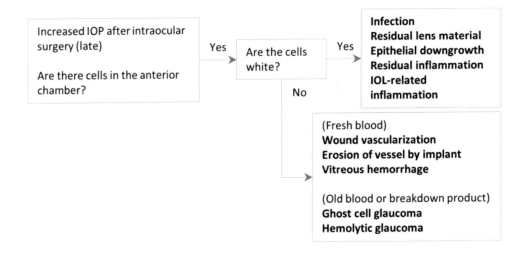

Later elevated IOP, no cells in the anterior chamber, open angle. If the patient is using corticosteroids, steroid-induced pressure elevation is a possibility. After discontinuing steroid use, the diagnostic possibilities are those discussed in Chapter 6. Occasionally open angle glaucoma develops after intraocular surgery and persists thereafter. We assume that damage to the outflow channels by the postoperative inflammation in individuals prone to chronic pressure elevation explains some episodes of elevated pressure that do not fall into other categories, although we cannot confirm this assumption.

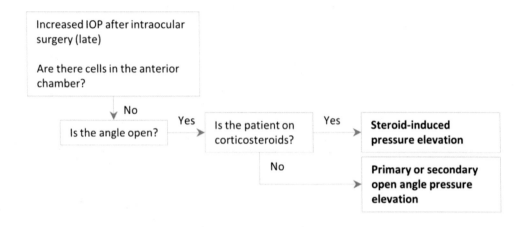

Later elevated IOP, no cells in the anterior chamber, closed angle. Residual PAS may result in chronic pressure elevation despite a patent iridotomy. This must be distinguished from currently active pupillary block, which may have persisted since surgery or may develop in the later postoperative period, particularly in individuals with anterior chamber lenses and in diabetic patients. Iris bombé is usually present in active pupillary block. If there is not a patent iridotomy, perform a laser iridotomy. Then evaluate and manage the patient as described in Chapter 9 for the management of patients with primary angle closure after relief of pupillary block. In a pseudophakic patient, if clinical exam cannot rule out the presence of a Soemmering's ring or retinal detachment, perform echography prior to doing an iridotomy. Iridotomy is contraindicated when the angle closure is attributed to an exuberant Soemmering's ring or total retinal detachment. Inadvertent puncturing of the Soemmering's ring capsule will allow hydration and expansion of retained cortical material and may result in anterior dislocation of the lens implant. Iatrogenic retinal perforation during iridotomy may occur in the setting of detached retina lying immediately posterior to the iridozonular diaphragm.

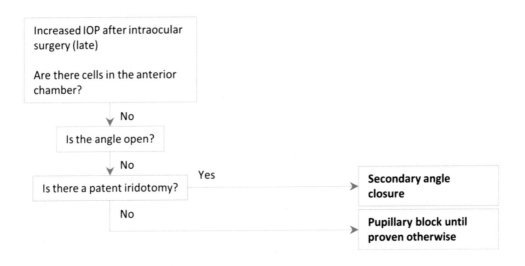

Elevated IOP Early after Blunt Trauma

Chart 11-3 summarizes our recommended approach to patients with high pressure after blunt trauma.

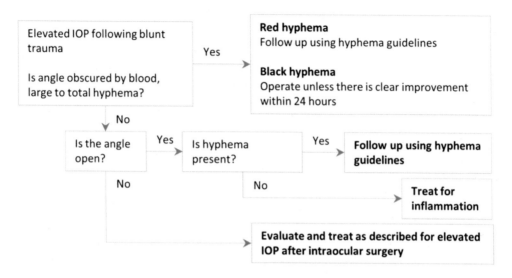

CHART 11-3. Diagnosis of high pressure following blunt trauma.

Elevated IOP, angle obscured by blood. We divide individuals with large to total hyphemas into two groups:

- Those with total or almost total red hyphemas with elevated pressure
- Those with total black hyphemas with elevated pressure

Total red hyphema and elevated pressure. Provided a total hyphema remains red, it almost always lyses within a fairly short period. We treat the eye as described for partial hyphema with two exceptions. The first is that early peripheral laser iridotomy is impossible, although with a total hyphema the likelihood of pupillary block is high. Until the clot contracts or begins to lyse, it is not possible to visualize the iris. Within a few days, the hyphema contracts and the peripheral iris becomes visible. If it is bowed forward, perform an iridotomy. The second difference in management is that we recommend surgery if the clot turns from red to black.

Total black hyphema and elevated pressure. Blood in the eye turns black when the red blood cells are concentrated and compacted by exit of serum. A black clot clears over an extended period, especially when aqueous flow through the anterior chamber is eliminated by pupillary block. When the pressure is elevated in such an eye, it has been our experience that the patient almost always develops either an afferent pupillary defect or corneal blood staining, usually after about a week. Therefore we now operate promptly unless there is a surgical contraindication or the patient's condition clearly improves within 24 hours. We perform a trabeculectomy and peripheral iridectomy. We may irrigate the anterior chamber gently, but we do not attempt to remove the clot because of the risks to the corneal endothelium and the chance of lens injury if the anterior segment is instrumented. To date, all the clots that we have treated in this manner have lysed and we have not had to reoperate to clear the hyphema.

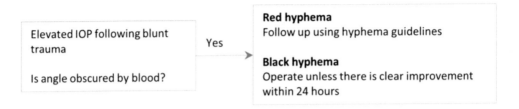

Elevated IOP, angle open, partial hyphema. Direct angle trauma, blockage of the trabecular meshwork by red blood cells, inflammation, and preexisting glaucoma may all contribute to elevated pressure. Because of the risk of recurrent bleeding, various regimens including bed rest, patching, and use of antifibrinolytics are recommended for treatment of hyphema.

Our routine treatment is as follows.

Medical management

- Shield the involved eye to prevent additional trauma.
- Treat with a long-acting cycloplegic agent (atropine or scopolamine twice daily) to pull the lens backward, to keep the ciliary muscle immobile, to decrease inflammation, and to relieve discomfort.
- Treat with corticosteroids at least four times a day to increase patient comfort, to decrease inflammation, and to retard synechiae formation.
- Treat with topical IOP-lowering medication (usually a beta-blocker) if the pressure is > 30 mmHg.
- Add an oral carbonic anhydrase inhibitor if the pressure is greater than 40 mmHg on topical treatment. We are aware of the concern that the use of carbonic anhydrase inhibitors in individuals with sickle cell trait and disease leads to acidosis and increased sickling. Current data neither confirm nor refute this possibility. We have used carbonic anhydrase inhibitors in individuals with sickle disease but routinely obtain medical consultation.
- Examine the patient daily and assess for an afferent defect daily using the consensual pupillary response.

Surgical treatment. Occasionally a patient with a partial hyphema and an initially open angle will develop pupillary block (from clot) and iris bombé that is clearly visible above the clot. Laser peripheral iridotomy resolves the bombé.

In a person with a partial hyphema, we do not routinely operate solely for hyphema-associated pressure unless one of the following is present:

- New development of an afferent defect
- Corneal blood staining

When surgery is performed, we perform a trabeculectomy and peripheral iridectomy and do not attempt to remove all the blood. The trabeculectomy allows a route for egress of blood, and the iridectomy relieves pupillary block. We expect that a filtering procedure done under these circumstances will fail within a fairly short period. We do not attempt to establish a long-term filtering procedure because of the risks associated with blebs and because of the usually transient nature of the early pressure elevations associated with hyphema.

Later treatment. Hyphemas generally clear within a few weeks. If the pressure remains elevated after the blood clears and the patient is no longer using corticosteroids, use the management regimen described on the next page.

Elevated IOP, angle open, no hyphema. Inflammation, direct trabecular meshwork damage, and preexisting glaucoma are the most likely possibilities in this situation. Treat the eye presumptively for inflammation and manage the pressure by the guidelines in Chapter 10 for a single episode of inflammation.

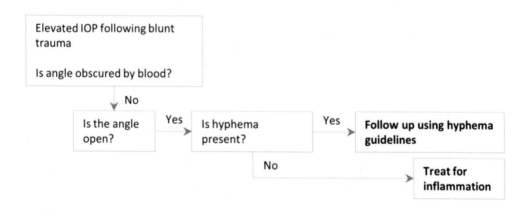

Elevated IOP, angle closed, with or without partial hyphema. The same general mechanisms of angle closure apply to accidental trauma as to surgical trauma. Once the angle is open, evaluate as previously described.

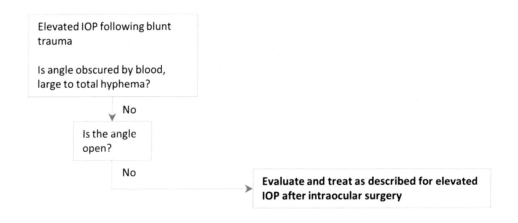

Persistent IOP Elevation after Blunt Trauma

Blunt trauma that responds to nonsurgical therapy, or at least is not severe enough to require prompt surgery, rarely causes elevated pressure that lasts longer than 1 or 2 months. If the pressure is still elevated 6 months after injury, and if the eye is not inflamed and no corticosteroids have been used for several weeks, establish a baseline for future follow-up of elevated pressure. The differences in the chronic management of elevated IOP related to blunt trauma compared with primary open angle pressure elevation are discussed in Chapter 12.

Elevated IOP after Intraocular Surgery – Special Considerations

Penetrating keratoplasty. Pupillary block may develop if no iridectomy is done at the time of the graft. Steroid-related pressure elevation often occurs after the first several weeks, and, if it develops, usually warrants treatment both because of the expected duration of the high pressure and because of the deleterious effect of elevated pressure on the corneal graft.

Filtering surgery. The following are the most common causes of high pressure immediately after filtering surgery:

- Tight closure of a scleral flap
- Blood under the scleral flap
- Internal blockage of the filtration ostium with blood, iris, lens, or vitreous
- Suprachoroidal hemorrhage with rotation of the iris and ciliary body and occlusion of the ostium

Pupillary block is uncommon because a peripheral iridectomy is usually performed, although recent variations in filtering procedures, especially use of a mini-shunt implant, do not include routine iridectomy. In these cases, pupillary block remains on the list of differential diagnoses. Ciliary block may develop, usually in eyes with previous angle closure. Hyphema, viscoelastic material, and direct trabecular meshwork damage do not raise the pressure in the presence of a functioning filtration bleb. Treatments are discussed in standard surgical texts. Later, fibrotic closure of the bleb (failure of the procedure) may result in pressure elevation.

Scleral buckle. Buckle-induced ciliary body rotation develops after scleral buckling procedures. The peripheral anterior chamber is usually flat and the central chamber is shallow. Peripheral iridotomy has not been successful in our experience, and we no longer perform it. The presumed pathophysiologic condition is forward rotation of the ciliary body and lens. Figure 11-8 illustrates the presumed mechanism. Our preferred treatment is iridoretraction (laser iridoplasty), accompanied by intense treatment with cycloplegics and corticosteroids.

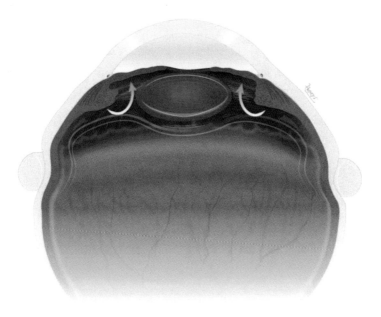

FIG. 11-8. Scleral buckle-induced angle closure. The ciliary body, lens and iris root rotate forward causing angle closure.

Pars plana vitrectomy with gas or silicone oil tamponade. A variety of gases remain in eyes after surgery. Some gases expand and some do not; all rise to the anterior part of the eye to block the pupil if the patient lies supine. A gas or silicone oil bubble that occludes the opening(s) between the anterior and posterior chambers causes pupillary block, apposition of the iris to the angle, and high pressure. If the patient is supine, a large bubble lies behind the pupil, but surface tension prevents it from entering the anterior chamber. As aqueous humor exits through the trabecular meshwork, the iris is lifted forward by the floating bubble until the anterior chamber is flat and the angle is closed. If an iridotomy is present and not covered by the bubble, the anterior chamber can flatten immediately because aqueous humor can pass posteriorly around the bubble and allow it to float anteriorly more freely. If the patient is sitting, the floating bubble can still flatten the anterior chamber if it is large enough (Fig. 11-9). Because eyes are often quite inflamed after procedures associated with gas or silicone oil bubbles, peripheral anterior synechiae may form rapidly. This condition warrants treatment if it is recognized. Face-down positioning of the patient and removal of some of the gas or silicone oil are options. Appropriate treatment should take into account both the effects of the pupillary block on the anterior segment and optic nerve and the condition for which the surgery was performed. A perfect IOP in an eye blinded by a retinal pathology does not benefit the patient.

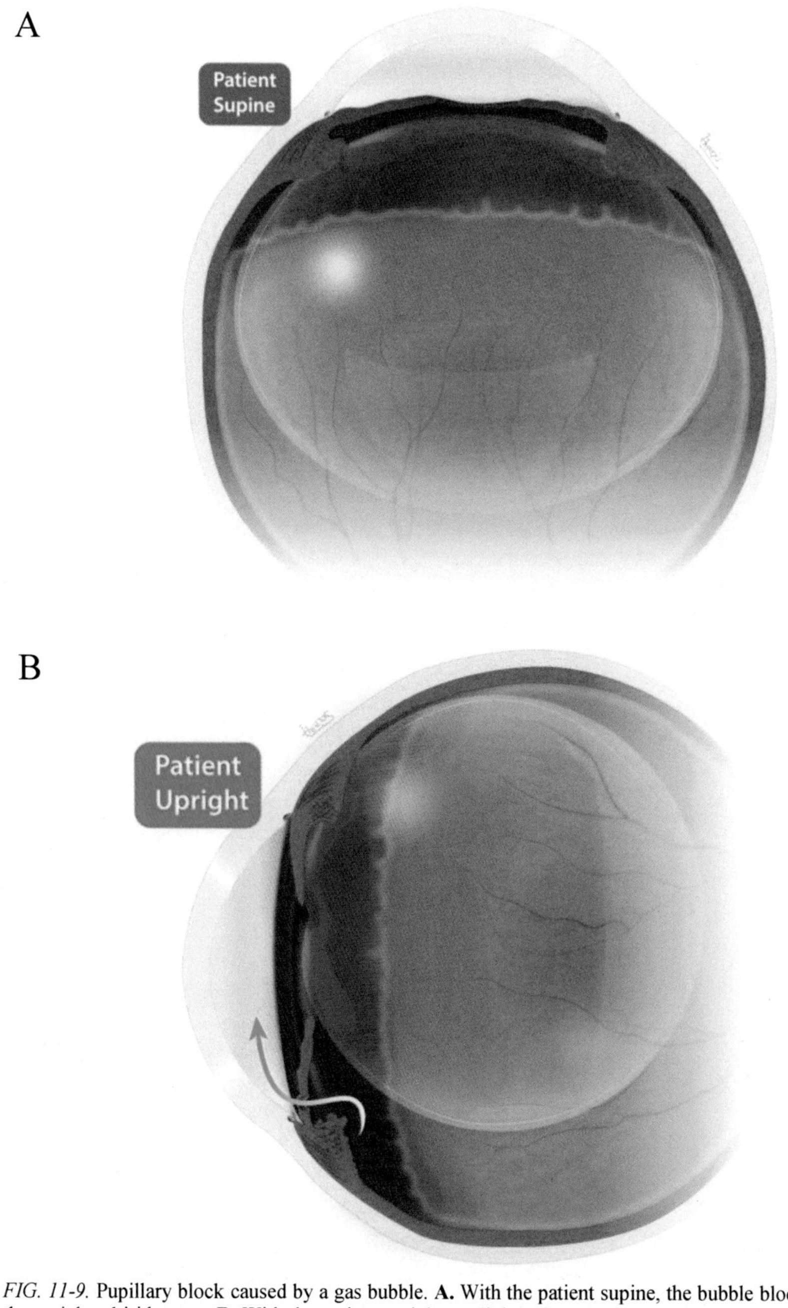

FIG. 11-9. Pupillary block caused by a gas bubble. **A.** With the patient supine, the bubble blocks both the pupil and the peripheral iridotomy. **B.** With the patient upright or slightly face-down, an inferior iridotomy allows aqueous to enter the anterior chamber and thus prevents pupillary block.

Reference

1. Kaplowitz K, Yung E, Flynn R, Tsai JC. Current concepts in the treatment of vitreous block, also known as aqueous misdirection. Survey of Ophthalmology. 2015 May-Jun;60(3):229-41.

12 MISCELLANEOUS CONDITIONS

This chapter discusses some of the particular differences of fairly common glaucomas from primary open angle glaucoma (POAG) in their care or in their usual course. It also describes an approach to patients who have strong family histories of glaucoma and to patients with large, but apparently normal, cups.

Pseudoexfoliation with Glaucoma

Pseudoexfoliation with open angle glaucoma differs from POAG in a few ways. Probably because the condition is associated with laxity of the zonules, angle closure develops in addition to open angle glaucoma more commonly than it does in POAG. Perform gonioscopy at least yearly and also promptly after adding miotic drops to the patient's treatment regimen. In our experience, patients with pseudoexfoliation have a tendency to develop rather abrupt increases in pressure even without angle closure. Thus a person whose intraocular pressure (IOP) has been well-controlled for years may develop a substantially increased pressure and may have symptoms of acutely elevated IOP. We therefore recommend that individuals with pseudoexfoliation and glaucoma be examined at least every 6 months. Patients with pseudoexfoliation usually respond well to laser trabeculoplasty.

Pigmentary Glaucoma

This condition is treated in the same manner as POAG. Patients with pigmentary glaucoma are often young and myopic. Miotics are effective in this condition, though the side effect of myopic shift, brow ache and the four times daily dosing may make compliance difficult. A randomized clinical trial was performed to determine if alleviating reverse pupillary block and irido-zonular chafing by laser iridotomy prevented pressure elevation in normotensive pigment dispersion patients. [1] In appropriate patients with pigment dispersion syndrome without glaucoma, we offer elective laser iridotomy.*

Elevated Episcleral Venous Pressure with Glaucoma

The glaucoma associated with high episcleral venous pressure, which may accompany cutaneous vascular malformation such as Sturge-Weber syndrome, responds poorly to medical and laser management because the resistance to outflow is beyond Schlemm's canal. We have had good success with incisional surgery in individuals with uncontrolled glaucoma and high episcleral venous pressure. Standard surgical texts describe the use of prophylactic

---

* In high risk patients, defined as those with at least 10 particles of pigment release in the anterior chamber after aggressive phenylephrine dilation (10% concentration, administered q5 minutes x 3), laser iridotomy decreased the 10-year incidence of a $\geq$ 5 mmHg IOP elevation from 61.9% (untreated group) to 14.3% (treated group). The clinical significance of this finding is uncertain, and the effect of laser iridotomy in manifest pigmentary glaucoma has not been evaluated.

sclerotomies in such cases, and we have followed these recommendations.

Glaucoma Associated with Blunt Trauma and Angle Recession

Acute high pressure after blunt trauma is described in Chapter 11. Glaucoma associated with trauma may also appear as an acute symptomatic elevated IOP as discussed in Chapter 9. The chronic pressure elevation that may follow blunt trauma is managed similarly to primary pressure elevation. Laser trabeculoplasty rarely lowers the pressure and sometimes results in increased pressure.

Steroid-Induced Pressure Elevation

Eliminating corticosteroid use, if possible, is the best treatment for steroid-induced pressure elevation. If this is not possible, steroid-induced pressure elevation from steroids used for nonocular conditions responds to medical, laser, and surgical therapies much as does primary open angle pressure elevation. If the steroids are used for ocular inflammation, the prognosis and treatment depend on the primary disease. Angle surgeries, such as goniotomy and trabeculotomy, work well in some patients with steroid induced pressure elevation.

Chronic Angle Closure Glaucoma

Primary chronic angle closure glaucoma usually presents as an asymptomatic pressure elevation. If the pressure decreases markedly after iridotomy, chronic management resembles that of primary acute angle closure after iridotomy (Chapter 9). In this circumstance, even if manifest glaucoma is present, the new IOP may generally be observed without treatment to determine whether it causes progressive glaucomatous damage.

If iridotomy does not alter the IOP significantly, the initial management and subsequent follow-up of chronic angle closure glaucoma differs little from that of open angle pressure elevation. The patient should have regular gonioscopic examinations to rule out angle narrowing related to anterior lens movement. Laser trabeculoplasty treatment is useful only in open areas of the angle.

Iridocorneal Endothelial Syndromes

The glaucoma associated with the iridocorneal endothelial syndromes is very difficult to treat and generally results in significant visual loss. There is no known treatment to halt the pathologic process, and the angle gradually closes. Laser trabeculoplasty is not effective, and many patients require surgery. As filtering procedures generally do not fare well, glaucoma drainage device implant procedures may have better outcomes.

Strong Family History of Open angle Glaucoma

A normotensive adult with a family history of severe glaucoma but no abnormal findings should have a yearly examination. We also obtain disc photos as a baseline record because the nerve appearance is less likely to change from a nonglaucomatous cause than is the field. If the pressure rises or the nerve appears to change, then we manage the condition by the routine guidelines in Chapters 2 through 5.

Large but Apparently Physiologic Cups

Sometimes a patient has large but healthy-looking cups – perhaps with large nerve heads – that do not appear glaucomatous and do not seem to warrant a major evaluation for glaucoma. The clinician should obtain optic disc photos, baseline optical coherence tomography of circumpapillary retinal nerve fiber layers, and a diagnostic field. If the visual field is normal, reexamine the patient periodically. Once progressive disease is ruled out, the patient is followed at routine intervals thereafter determined by the patient's age.

Reference

1. Gandolfi SA, Ungaro N, Tardini MG, Ghirardini S, Carta A, Mora P. A 10-year follow-up to determine the effect of YAG laser iridotomy on the natural history of pigment dispersion syndrome: a randomized clinical trial. JAMA Ophthalmology. 2014 Dec;132(12):1433-8

INDEX

ABOUT THE AUTHORS

Ta Chen Peter Chang (tachenchang@hotmail.com) received his medical training at the Johns Hopkins School of Medicine. After an ophthalmology residency at Stanford University, he completed a glaucoma fellowship at the Bascom Palmer Eye Institute in Miami, Florida, and a pediatric ophthalmology fellowship at Vanderbilt University in Nashville, Tennessee. He is a faculty member of the Bascom Palmer Eye Institute with clinical and research interests in glaucoma, cataract and strabismus in both adults and children.

Pradeep Ramulu received his medical degree at the Johns Hopkins School of Medicine and stayed on to complete his residency at the Johns Hopkins Wilmer Eye Institute. He completed his glaucoma fellowship at the Bascom Palmer Eye Institute, and then returned to Johns Hopkins to join the Wilmer faculty, where he splits his time researching the impact of glaucoma on the person and providing clinical and surgical care to glaucoma patients.

Elizabeth Hodapp graduated from Harvard Medical School. She completed her ophthalmology residency and glaucoma fellowship at Washington University in St. Louis. She serves on the faculty at the Bascom Palmer Eye Institute and treats adult and children with glaucoma.

Illustrator

Aristomenis Thanos (aristhanos@gmail.com) completed his medical education at the National Kapodistrian University of Athens, Greece, followed by ophthalmology residency training at the Massachusetts Eye & Ear Infirmary. He is currently a vitreoretinal fellow at Associated Retinal Consultants, William Beaumont Hospital. His medical illustrations, primarily in the field of ophthalmology, have been featured in several scientific journals and textbooks.